ALWAYS STAY YOUNG

The secret to living long

Lola Steven

used only for reference. No endorsement is implied when we use one of these terms.

Don't be afraid to grow old. Getting older is not a disease. Aging is the most beautiful phase of life, the one in which you have the opportunity to take things lightly and see reality from the best perspective. So face aging with the right spirit and the right allies to live a long and healthy life!

I like to imagine myself old with my grandchildren and still smart while I exercise, attend conferences, take courses, swim, dedicate time to discover new places, being together with my loved ones. A simple world, made of simple things, full of joy, surrounded by people with whom to share a part of life, but who is active, until the light goes out.

What about you? How do you see yourselves in twenty or thirty years or more?

I believe that this book can help you to kindle hope, not to complain about your age, the ailments we all have, but to dedicate time to improve yourself also learning some advice from our oriental friends, where serious diseases and low longevity are rare events.

So if before now you imagined yourself in a rocking chair as an elderly, scrutinizing the clouds, the stars, motionless and waiting for your hour, know that this book in small but constant steps will overturn your way of thinking or saying: "I am old, I am fifty years old".

I want to imagine you all as a bright dragon that slowly but steadily moves in the world, happy because every day it has learned something new, inspired by the many ideas and experiences that will surely come to mind reading the next chapters.

I anticipate what the topics will be and in summary my way of seeing life and my world.

In fact, I am pleased to share my journey with my many readers.

AGEING

Let's start right away with the hottest topic.

What happens to the epidermis after the age of fifty? It becomes thin and shows pigmentation alterations that reduce resistance to light, the dermis becomes less elastic, hair thins and thins, nails become thin, the inflammatory and immune response is altered, bone density is reduced, weakening of the skeleton causes changes in the face, jaw and lower limbs. Other changes affect the spine and cause a reduction in stature. The older you get, the harder it is to lose your accumulated weight, because your metabolism and physical activity tend to decrease with increasing age. The respiratory system suffers the consequences of aging due to the weakening of the respiratory organs, overeating generates diabetes and hypertension. The time of onset of arteriosclerosis is shortened. With increasing age, the number of nerve cells decreases and brain weight decreases by 10% each year.

Up to the age of seventy a reduction in vocabulary richness can be observed, a slower slowness in carrying out daily tasks and some memory lapse may occur.[1]

After describing all that we will lose over the years, let's figure out how to preserve what we have.

---

[1] Source: Johns Hopkins, *The Johns Hopkins Medical Guide to Health After 50*, Black Dog & Leventhal, New York, 2006.

SLOWING DOWN AGING: THE SECRETS TO STAYING YOUNG AND HEALTHY

Free radicals

Biological age is closely linked to the levels of oxidative stress of our cells, or oxidative substances that literally attack our body. If we age faster, free radicals are to blame, the main responsible for damage to our skin, thinning hair and the appearance of degenerative diseases such as atherosclerosis. In short, real enemies of our aesthetic appearance and our health!

Free radicals are substances produced during energy processes in which oxygen is used. We could define them as a waste product of metabolism. If our body produces it in high quantities, a situation of oxidative stress is created that causes real cellular damage. Free radicals affect every cell in our body and can cause reversible or irreversible damage to proteins, nucleic acids and lipids.

If a certain amount of free radicals is to be considered physiological, their increase can be the consequence of conditions such as:

1. overweight;

2. prolonged psychophysical stress;

3. exposure to environmental pollution;

4. Unbalanced diet too high in fat and low in fiber.

All these factors should be eliminated to stay young and full of energy longer!

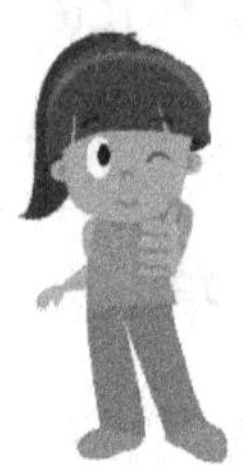

"Youth is happy, because it has the ability to see beauty. Anyone who retains the ability to capture beauty will never grow old."

FRANZ KAFKA

Antioxidants: friends for the skin

But how to intervene to bring the situation back into balance, eliminate oxidative stress and slow down aging?

Simple, since free radicals are nothing more than waste substances, the best thing we can do is wipe them out. And here comes antioxidants, sworn enemies of free radicals. The most well-known antioxidants are vitamin E and vitamin C.

These substances help our body to get rid of waste produced during metabolic processes and reduce the negative effects caused by free radicals.

Foods rich in antioxidants are carrots, tomatoes, fruit, spinach, chard, green leafy vegetables and whole grains.

Healthy habits to stay young longer

In addition to a healthy and balanced diet, physical exercise, allowing yourself moments of rest and relaxation, cultivating your interests, sleeping an adequate number of hours, limiting alcohol consumption and eliminating smoking can be a very valuable aid to combat premature aging and stay young. In addition, if you really want to do good for the skin, limit sun exposure.

Excessive exposure to UVA and UVB rays accelerates the aging processes of the skin, especially for lighter phototypes, present to a lesser extent than darker complexions , which are more vulnerable to damage from excessive tanning.

Sunburned skin is and will remain an injured skin forever, even if you have subsequently used repairing creams or after sun. To prevent premature aging of the skin it is therefore a good idea to keep away from too intense sun exposure and remember that when you want to tan you should use a good sunscreen.

It is useful to maintain a good intellectual activity by leading a life full of interests. Spending large sums on aesthetic beauty care does not improve the function of the most important organs for the quality of our life.

Interventions are needed to slow down biological aging and delay the onset of diseases of old age.

To live all human beings need energy and most of it is obtained from the oxidation of food.

About 1% of the oxygen we consume produces free radicals that attack cells and damage them. In addition, sugars can also damage the molecules of our cells and cause alterations in collagen.

It has been shown that fasting one day a week extends life by almost 50%.

Many restricted diet animals enjoy excellent health until old age. In addition, physical activity has significant beneficial effects, many animals raised in cages equipped for physical activity and who are subjected to a caloric restriction diet live longer.

If you want to get the maximum benefit, life must be active, rich in intellectual stimuli but you have to limit stress.

In animals, these interventions prolong life and reduce all diseases associated with old age. With a varied diet, rich in fish, vegetables, fresh and dried fruits, the use of supplements should not be necessary except in old age.

Over the age of seventy there is often a deficiency of vitamin B6 and B12, folic acid, vitamin D, E, calcium. In particular, the desire for sweet and savoury foods for diabetes and blood pressure must be resisted, and I will explain why in more detail later.

300 grams of cold-water fish, such as salmon and blue fish, and nuts can be useful to our body together with fruits, vegetables and foods rich in bran. A short but constant period of fasting increases cell turnover and promotes the renewal and rejuvenation of the quality of life.

Physical exercise is one of the most effective systems to increase lifespan, walking for example for six, seven kilometers a day allows muscle turnover, determined by the repair of microtraumas of the fibers.

Sleep disorders should be resolved through the use of melatonin late in the evening.[2]

So dietary restrictions and mild pharmacological interventions allow to amplify the benefits to counteract aging and prevent diseases of old age.

Enduring the sense of hunger for a few hours is a sign that the body is cleaning itself of all harmful waste, while following a healthy diet rich in fruits and vegetables and some multivitamins helps longevity.

Being overweight is dangerous, because it slows down the turnover of cellular

---

[2] E. J. Masoro, *Caloric restriction: a key to understanding and modulating aging, Volume 1,* Elsevier Science, Amsterdam 2002.; G. S. Roth, M. A. LAne D. K. Ingram, *Biomarkers of caloric restriction may predict longevity in humans in science,* 297, pp. 811-2002.

structures and is second only to smoking among the avoidable causes of death. Those who smoke a pack of cigarettes a day have a risk of developing heart failure, while drinking a glass of wine, a liqueur a day is an acceptable habit In addition, sun exposure should be avoided during aging, because pigmentation tends to decrease with increasing age.

Positive social interactions are important because they lower plasma levels of stress hormones and prevent depression.

As I said, with the passing of the years the short memory diminishes and the reaction times lengthen and therefore it takes more time to assimilate new information, even if learning new things is very important.

As we have said, eating well is the most powerful method against aging. In addition, with age the ability to absorb and use some nutrients is reduced and it is advisable to consume diets richer in antioxidants such as fruits, vegetables, cereals, avoiding red meats, whole dairy products, butter, coconut oil, packaged foods, using olive oil and to a lesser extent sunflower or corn oil and consuming salmon, tuna and sardines.

Limit the use of salt for hypertension and consume vegetables of dark green or orange color. As drinks, drink at least eight glasses of water a day and alternate moments of intense calorie restriction with moments of overeating, where you will have to feel hungry to then recover the mass lost after fasting.

Hunger is a signal that tells us that our cells are getting rid of broken and aged components and preparing space for new and functioning components.

What physical activity exercises should I do? Aerobic activities such as running or cycling, which stress the cardiovascular system, and strength exercises with the use of light weights and stretching, we also recommend a thirty-minute walk at a brisk pace three times a week.

What are the benefits of walking? In addition to the vascular system, the functionality of the heart, lungs and bones is helped. Walking even protects against diseases such as Alzheimer's and helps regulate blood pressure. Older adults who exercise accumulate less fat than sedentary peers, increasing good cholesterol.

Aerobic activities that help are walking, climbing stairs, which help strengthen bones and improve leg muscle strength. Swimming is also a recommended activity. Finally, sport increases self-esteem, which is essential protection against depression.

Regular exercise improves mental faculties, including memory. Stretching improves balance, posture and sensitivity to fatigue and pain, reducing anxiety and optimizing breathing rate.

Among supplements, resveratrol can be very helpful in neutralizing free radicals before they can damage cells.

Some studies on populations that feed on diets rich in fish and Omega 3 show that the subjects examined enjoy a long and healthy life and its administration can counteract oxidative stress and promote health and longevity.

We know that 61% of Americans are overweight or obese, and it is worrying that obesity is increasing in all segments of the population, including children, as we now have unprecedented amounts of cheap food and eat more than we need.

On the calorie ratio, we should record in a diary the values of food and activities to understand how much we dedicate to physical exercise and how we eat, setting a limit to fats and oils, burgers and fries, especially in the afternoon. Regardless of age, those suffering from hypertension, liver disease, kidney disease or heart failure should refrain from alcohol consumption.

So what is the elixir of life?

The human being is always looking for something that gives beauty, youth and long life, but we are witnessing a reduction in health, especially in recent years, where people live more but without fully enjoying well-being. I advise you then to let yourself go on this journey for the future and for your health.

In my life, volleyball has been my salvation, because dedicating myself only to study I had reduced relationships with others, I had closed in on myself in my world made of books and art.

Instead, thanks to a friend who enrolled me in these courses without telling me, I managed to anchor myself firmly to my closest friends and I lived the best years of adolescence without ever stopping playing. Volleyball teaches you discipline, rules and respect for the opponent.

Team spirit makes you full of energy for the benefit of the whole team. I must say that sport has given me so much, having had problems with wrong nutrition during my adolescence.

I discovered how proper nutrition allows you to have more energy and to carry out all the activities of the day.

Here in the book you will find useful information and recipes for a long life.

Have you ever wondered how balanced your diet can be?

And how much rest per day?

What is your current state of well-being and your work productivity?

Have you ever wondered how important relationships and the time you devote to hobbies and entertainment?

Improvement is necessary for all of us and allows a general well-being.

Starting with a positive day allows us to access the full potential of our energy resources, while the effect of a sedentary lifestyle causes many more deaths than tumors. 80% percent of our health depends on us and our daily choices.

It is time to act now. As far as physical exercise is concerned, we can always be accompanied by an expert trainer, who will be able to indicate a personalized training scheme.

If we also want to eat better, we can rely on a good nutritionist, who will allow us to make a tailor-made path with a diet suitable for our BMI (Body Mass Index).

A balanced diet must be maintained throughout life, without using junk foods and without exceeding sugar and salt.

Clearly you can always use a day dedicated to the vices that will not compromise the results achieved, instead eating in excess increases blood sugar, makes the pancreas produce an excessive amount of insulin which then determines a glycemic drop that causes a feeling of hunger, fatigue and drowsiness.

The consumption of fruit in the morning helps the body to purify, but it is good to understand how.

To take the fats necessary for the body we recommend the use of extra virgin olive oil and the consumption of dried fruit and pumpkin seeds in moderation, while consuming more carbohydrates especially when doing sports can help in terms of energy to move.

Finally, proteins are also important, which are used to keep our muscle structure healthy and strong.

In this regard, the consumption of white meat is useful, limiting that of red meat and sausages. Eggs are also an excellent source of protein. Other foods that contribute to our well-being are rice milk, coconut milk, chicken cold cuts, protein bars, biscuits with rye, oats, kamut, buckwheat, spelled and rice pasta.

The use of coffee must be limited and, as already mentioned, fasting has countless health benefits since autophagy is a mechanism of cell cleansing.

Autophagy is accentuated in case of energy deficiency, therefore eating less and fasting.

In addition, I recommend the importance of ionotherapy, which takes place by means of ionized water of which I spoke in another book of mine.

This book invites you to cultivate your passions, to focus on what you love to do.

"In the world nothing great has been done without   passion."
GEORG WILHELM FRIEDRICH HEGEL

A MEANINGFUL LIFE HELPS TO LIVE LONG

What motivates people every day is to live according to their *mission*. This is a question I've always asked myself: why am I in the world? What is my role in the world?

I came across some books on *ikigai,* the definition of which is rather complex. *Ikigai* is the goal that a person sets for which it is worth getting up in the morning. It answers the question: Why am I here? What is the meaning of my life? Iwant to share with you my *ikigai,* which is to help others improve. Since I graduated, my goal has always been this, in every society, in every situation, and when I didn't the results were bad. *Ikigai* prolongs life. People who get up every morning with a specific goal give meaning to their existence and live longer.

The philosophy of *ikigai* originated in Japan in 794 and developed until 1185. It found its diffusion in 1966 thanks to the publication of the book *ikigai* on the meaning of life by the Japanese psychiatrist Mieko Kamiya.

Akihiro Asegawa, a clinical psychologist, introduced *ikigai* into the Japanese language in 2001 and it was later discovered that it was one of the secrets of the extraordinary longevity of the population of the island of Okinawa.

Knowing the purpose of one's life and the value of one's uniqueness is the beginning of our emotional healing and our psychophysical health.

To find *Ikigai* it is necessary to undergo an aptitude test and when we accurately identify our *ikigai*, it is forever. The meaning of our life is to find our gift to give it to others. The moment we find our *Ikigai*, everyone can recognize himself in his truest essence. *Ikigai* is used as an effective method of selection and training of personnel to build motivated and efficient work teams.

What changes in our lives when we find *ikigai*? Everything, because from that moment we understand what is really essential for us and we stop being useless to ourselves turning into a real gift.

To find *ikigai* it is necessary to undergo an aptitude test available on the www.professionistaper.com/ikigaihappiness website, containing the questions mentioned here and the reference to the specific book. Through the outcome of the test, you will have a spurt in your evolutionary growth and everything will make sense. The questions are 56 and below I propose some that can be important to get your *ikigai.* For each you will have to strive to give at least three answers:

- What am I passionate about talking to my friends at length?

- I have a whole day off, how would I like to spend it?

- What are the things people or circumstances that charge me with energy?

- What are the things I do with the most pleasure?

- For what qualities do I most often receive compliments or praise?

- What am I willing to do even for free just for the pleasure of doing it?

- What do the world and humanity need most?

At the end of the questionnaire you will find the word that summarizes all the information you have previously grouped.

"*About life more than its logic, only then will you understand its meaning.*"
DOSTOEVSKY

"*To be what we are, to become what we are capable of becoming, this is the only purpose of life.*"
ROBERT LOUIS STEVENSON

ACCEPT WHAT WE ARE

Acceptance of what we are and those around us (family, colleagues...) allows us to live better.

By accepting others we will also be able to understand their point of view, which may be different from ours, but we will want to understand it without judging it. And it is when you come to this acceptance that you are able to make a change in various situations, going to eliminate stress. We must become aware of what is happening around us and accept it as it is. Change should not be seen as something negative, but as something natural. Once you have the opportunity to calmly observe what surrounds you, understanding the point of view of others, you will have more power over your emotions. This will allow you to connect better with yourself to renewvi, as nature itself does. All this effort willmake **positive changes in the person's body**: it regulates blood pressure and reduces the impact of stress.

One must accept circumstances and **learn** to **be useful both to oneself and to others**.

THE IMPORTANCE OF GLUCOSE

What is glucose?

What are spikes and why are they harmful?

What can we do to avoid them while continuing to eat our favorite foods?

After the launch of the "23andme" project, professional athletes started wearing CGMs (Continuous Glycemic Monitoring), using glucose level measurement to optimize performance and endurance. Some scientific articles have demonstrated the usefulness of these devices to detect regular glucose levels even in non-diabetic subjects.

In the book *The Glucose Revolution*, author Jessie Inchaus conducted experiments noting everything that happened. The kitchen was his laboratory, his hypothesis was that food and movement influenced glucose levels according to precise rules. Where should we start?

We must start from glucose, because among all the levers that our body possesses, glucose is the onewith the greatest effect on our well-being. In fact, it immediately influences the way we feel, since it affects hunger and mood and, once we have it under control, glucose triggers a positive domino effect. If blood sugar levels are imbalanced, the lights come on, the alarms sound, we gain weight, the hormones are out of control, we feel tired and we want sugar, the skin suffers, the heart suffers and we risk developing diabetes. According to a recent theory, when mitochondria are overwhelmed by excess glucose, small molecules are released that have important consequences, free radicals. These molecules are harmful, because they damage everything they touch, modify the points in random points of our genetic code, creating mutations that activate harmful genes that can cause a tumor. When we fail to neutralize free radicals, the body is subjected to a condition of oxidative stress that contributes to the onset of heart disease and cognitive decline. Fructose increases it even more than glucose, it is one of the reasons why sweets that contain fructose are worse for health than foods that do not contain it. Fat-free processed foods actually contain a lot of sucrose and this means that fructose is transformed into fat after digestion.

Are you always hungry? It is a symptom of elevated insulin levels. The answer is not to try to eat less, but to reduce insulin levels. Each spike worsens the long-term abilities of the mitochondria and leads to greater fatigue. Of all the organs, the brain is the one that requires the most energy. It houses a lot of mitochondria and if excess glucose occurs, the brain can suffer the consequences. Repeated glycemic peaks promote the onset of neuroinflammation and cognitive dysfunction. Those who adopt a diet that causes irregular glucose levels report worse mood, more depressive symptoms and greater malaise.

Here in the book the author talks about how to eat foods in the right order.

According to a famous article from Corner University in 2015 ("Diabetes Care" 38,n.7,2015 e98-e99), eating the foods of a meal in a specific order can reduce the peak of glucose by 73% and insulin by 48%. But what is the right order? First the fibers must be taken, then proteins and fats, finally starches and sugars. The discovery was sensational. If starch or sugars enter the stomach first, they pass quickly into the intestine giving rise to a peak. Fiber, on the other hand, slows gastric emptying and flattens the glucose curve, the sugar starches that we ingest after fiber will therefore have a reduced effect on the body, so the right order will be vegetables first, then proteins, fats and finally carbohydrates, the slower glucose is absorbed by the blood the flatter our curve will be and the pancreas will produce less insulin.

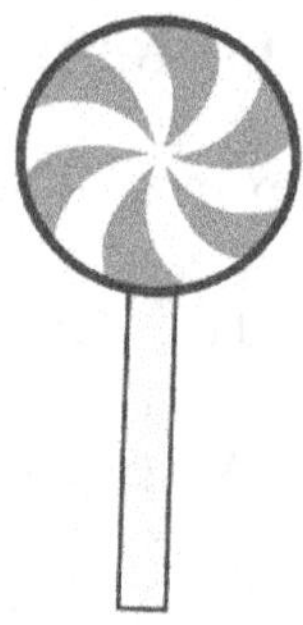

"*Passion can have a thousand different forms but its purpose is always the same: to make us feel alive.*"

FABRIZIO CARAMAGNA

THE BENEFITS OF EXERCISE

A study of 10,000 adolescents showed the link between exercise and positive self-image. The more sporty the boys, the happier and more balanced they are and have fewer problematic behaviors.

The answers are all within us, so let's start by identifying our main goal and intermediate goals, even writing a small diary, noting the days in which you will do gymnastics, the schedules, the days. Start progressively with constancy better little than nothing and reward yourself and gratify yourself to celebrate your successes. And here your elixir of life is ready.

The use of pilates was also very useful in my sporting activity, which looks a bit like yoga, but which allows you to activate all parts of the body. Below I propose an example of pilates scheme as a virtuous circle for our well-being.

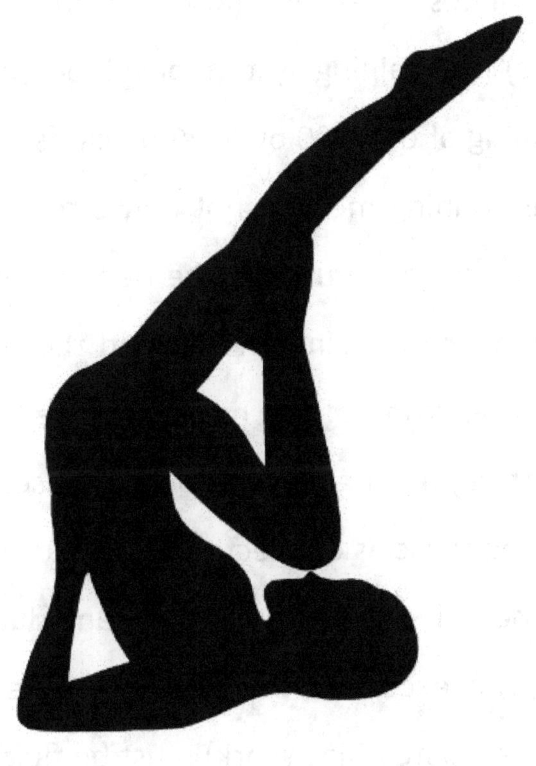

Pilates Method

The Pilates Method (also called simply Pilates) is a training system developed at the beginning of the '900 by Joseph Pilates.

This training method not only strengthens the abdominals, but also the deeper muscle bands near the spine and around the pelvis. The cornerstone of the method is the toning and strengthening of the Power House, that is, all the muscles connected to the trunk: the abdomen, buttocks, adductors and lumbar area. The exercises that are performed on the mat (Pilates Mat Work) must be fluid and perfectly executed, and must also be combined with correct breathing.

Pilates, if practiced regularly, has numerous benefits: it improves coordination and breathing, develops muscle and cardiovascular tone, is useful for concentration, defines the muscles and moisturizes the fascial tissues.

The 8 fundamental principles of the Pilates Method

The original Pilates method has no registration mark, so every teacher with the necessary preparation of physical motor education and postural principles can bring him closer to his style (see the Postural Pilates method) and his personality, but he must refer to the basic principles of Pilates:

1. BREATHING; always well controlled and guided by the help of the teacher, as in the practice of yoga (specifically in Pilates you breathe in starting the exercise and at the time of greater effort you

exhale, unlike yoga, you inhale with your nose and exhale both with the nose and with the mouth and for each exercise you adopt a precise rhythm);

2. the CENTER of GRAVITY; synonymous with Power House, it is seen as a center of strength and control of the whole body;

3. PRECISION; every movement must approach perfection, a closed-circuit work where the teacher must have continuous feedback from the student;

4. CONCENTRATION; maximum attention and concentration in each exercise, the mind must be the supervisor for every single part of the body;

5. CONTROL; it must take place on every part of the body, thoughtless and neglected movements must not be made;

6.   FLUIDITY; principle that is the synthesis of all the previous concepts. In its most sublime form, Pilates is "poetry in motion" (page 12 of the book "" by);[3]

7.   ISOLATION; mental concentration on exercise leads to dissecting our body through the work of isolation of some deep muscle groups, compared to others;

8.   the ROUTINE; The will and constancy in the practice of discipline make the difference.

I have always been struck by Japan, which has enormous knowledge about health, relationships and kindness. The Academic

[3] Alycea Ungaro, *Pilates, the promise of a new body,* Fabbri, Milan, 2005, p. 12.

Health Organization estimates a depression rate of 7% in Japan. In America this figure stands at 19%. The difference lies in their outlook on life. For the Japanese population it is not important to be happy, but to live with disappointment, to make others happy, even a loss must be accepted, compared to the American individualistic vision. When we accept the other and feel close to him, we create a greater chance of feeling good.

Who am I? The goal for the Japanese people must not be human selfishness. I am the one who can make things better.

The inhabitants of Okinawa, for example, almost never contract pathological diseases such as diabetes or cancer, they use a technique that is *kaizen*, that is, continuous change to always improve in all aspects of personal life and relationships at work both for themselves and for others.

They verify the results, analyze what they have achieved and make a change. In fact, if after making a mistake you do nothing to change you continue to fail.

Once the list has been compiled, we must be aware of the presence of mistakes, of the less beautiful aspects of our personality, and adopt attitudes aimed at improving them as well as being aware of our strengths. We must regularly dedicate hours to training and skills that make us more special. In addition , you have to take care of the body through nutrition.

We are what we eat, but not only what we eat, also how we eat it. If we eat 80% of what we need our digestion will be faster and our organs will work much better without having feelings of fatigue and weight conserving a greater amount of energy and we will feel more active.

Of course, we will not be able to imitate all the Japanese habits because they have many customs, but continuous physical activity is an excellent routine, in fact they take care of the housework, cultivate the garden every day, write a diary every morning and always keep busy. They feel they are the messenger, they ask themselves the question: how do we solve the problem? You and the other person are on the same side, face the situation together so the goals will be in common. How did you fix the problem earlier? Have you ever had a similar situation?

In this way I learn to accept the other. Or serving the other a little more and feeling what he feels in his heart, will help you to calm stress and anger. This will push you beyond happiness.

Exercise also promotes the production of endorphins, the feeling of happiness and prevents cognitive impairment. The joy of sharing and the satisfaction you feel in helping others are important. First well-being must be created, the point of view of the other must be understood, accepting one's family, one's colleagues and with the calm obtained one will be able to face the problems that have caused sadness.

"A lonely man is something imperfect, he must find a second one to be happy."
BLAISE PASCAL

"Loneliness is very beautiful... when you have someone close to you to tell it."
GUSTAVO ADOLFO BÉCQUER

A HINT OF EMOTIONAL HEALING: NEGATIVE ION THERAPY

As a naturopath I use the beneficial action of negative ions and the energy they transmit to the body as a real preventive therapy for my clients.

A client of mine, Luisa, told me that after the treatment she wakes up rested and energetic, also finding an incredible analgesic effect.

Health lies in a state of bioelectric balance that must be maintained both at the cellular and extracellular level. With the contribution of the Nobel Prize for Physics, Antoine Henri Becquerel, it has been highlighted that the human body is electrified for the most part of negative charge and that when this becomes insufficient the body is weakened.

The vitality of the organism depends precisely on the negative charge and when its relationship with the positive one is unbalanced, the state of health has a decompensation.

Subsequent studies have made it possible to understand how it is possible to act in depth, activating the natural self-repair processes within the body to the advantage of rapid and stable results over time.

There are several devices that send negative ions directly to the heart of the cells, bringing significant benefits to the overall health of the person. By introducing negative ions it is in fact possible to obtain the rebalancing of intra and extracellular homeostasis.

This therapy can be used to treat mood imbalances and in these years of pandemic I have faced many such cases.

The first studies on the benefits of negative ions on mood disorders date back to 1998 and have multiplied since then.

The results show that increased exposure to both negative ions and bright light helps alleviate these disorders, promoting a greater balance of mood.

It is the same that you feel standing in front of the waves of the sea and breathing these ions or diving in mountain waterfalls. The body regenerates.

The therapy is also very useful for insomnia and other sleep disorders that are becoming very common. The latest research shows that among the causes of insomnia is an imbalance in serotonin production. The negative ions intervene in the rebalancing of this neurotransmitter thus improving the quality of sleep.

"*It is the soul that you must change, not the sky under which you live!*"
LUCIUS ANNEUS SENECA

"*When I'm healthy, music drips from my fingers.*"
GEORGE GERSHWIN

HOW OLD DO YOU THINK YOU ARE?

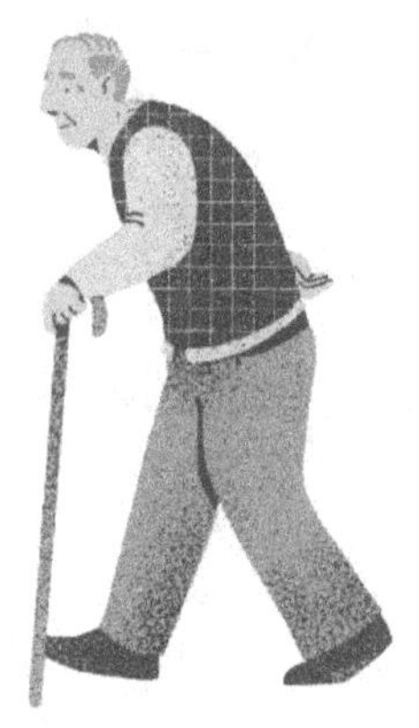

Many people think that ten extra pounds is not a problem and that sports is the stuff of fanatics.

Yet the recipe against premature aging has long been known: it is called a correct lifestyle.

Let's start by saying that there are two different ages: the registry and the biological. The chronological age is what we really have; The biological age is instead what our organs and our systems demonstrate. To give a better idea, let's take a fifty-year-old woman as an example. Its organs and systems can be: in line with its age; In better conditions they may be more functional than those of a younger woman. Each of us, therefore, can age prematurely, or on the contrary slow down this process.

How to slow down premature aging? Today's life puts a strain on our body: too much stress, unbalanced diet, air pollution, sedentary lifestyle, excess alcohol and drugs, smoking. These factors contribute to damage our body, causing us to lose health and leading us to have a biological age higher than we would physiologically have.

Outward appearance (fitness, wrinkles, etc.) is the most obvious consequence of premature aging, a factor that also increases the risk of contracting diseases and worsens the quality of life. To stay fit, keep us as healthy as possible, it is good to reverse the course and adopt a correct lifestyle, eliminating everything that hurts us.

Our goal must above all be health, also improving good mood and quality of life.

We often talk about free radicals, but do we really know them?

These molecules, enemies of cells, are waste that is formed mainly during energy production.

A high amount of free radicals damages our cells to the point of destroying them, triggering dangerous reactions such as: the acceleration of cellular aging processes and the risk of arteriosclerosis; However, we can make sure that they do not multiply by eating in the right quantities and adopting a correct lifestyle.

The production of free radicals is in fact accelerated by smoking, alcohol, intake of toxic substances, pollution, long exposure to the sun, excessive physical activity. Fortunately, our body develops systems of protection from the effects of free radicals.

The function of antioxidants is to fight free radicals so that they do not harm our cells. Antioxidants are friends of our cells, of our well-being and help to slow down the aging of our body. Some vitamins and minerals, flavonoids and other trace elements are antioxidants. We find them in many foods, both in the plant world (such as fruit, vegetables, legumes) and in the animal world (such as milk and dairy products, fish, eggs, etc.). The best way to take all the antioxidants that our body needs is to follow a balanced diet, which leads us to consume numerous foods particularly rich in protective substances.

The rules to counteract aging with nutrition are:

- eats five meals a day, three main meals (breakfast, lunch and dinner) and two snacks;

- Protect your cells: introduce fish (fresh or frozen) at least twice a week. Give preference to cod, because it is rich in polyunsaturated fatty acids that, among other benefits, lower cholesterol and prevent strokes and other cardiovascular diseases. Omega 3 are also present in other foods such as dried fruit (walnuts, almonds, pumpkin seeds, etc.);

- counteracts free radicals: consume two portions of vegetables daily, preferring raw ones to cooked ones, remembering that the former better maintain their beneficial properties against free radicals;

- Defend your body: consume fruit in snacks. The vitamin C contained in many fruits (citrus fruits, cherries, strawberries, kiwis, etc.) stimulates the immune system and reduces the risk of infections;

- Take all the antioxidants: vary the colors of vegetables and fruit throughout the week or even better every day;

- Strengthen your body: consume a semi-skimmed yogurt or skimmed milk every day. These dairy products provide good amounts of vitamin A, E, zinc, selenium and other important minerals, especially calcium, which defend and the body;

- Improve your health: use extra virgin olive oil, preferably raw, because it is rich in monounsaturated fatty acids. These nutrients improve the health of cells and the organism, preventing from certain types of cancer and other diseases;

- reduce salt consumption;
- hydrates your body;

- Push away what hurts you: only very rarely drink sugary drinks. Limit wine to 1-2 glasses per day.

"As we get older, you lose a lot of things that we didn't know we had."
CARLO GRAGNANI

"In youth the days are short and the years are long; In old age the years are short and the days are long."
NIKITA PANIN IVANOVICH

"Old age is life in slow motion. Because of this, the elderly see better."

THEODOR CODREANU

CONCLUSIONS

No excuses, start today!

The United States ranks 35th for life expectancy, Japan is in 2nd place. We look and learn from those who do better than us.

We learn to understand that the path to health and well-being is a journey in search of ourselves and the positive effects deriving from our healthier behaviors and helps us not to be alone, even doing outdoor activities together with others, listening to nature and talking less. Feel something that makes you feel useful.

It can be useful to keep a food diary for example by writing down what you eat and how many antioxidants you take.

"Be the _change_ *you would like to see* _happen_ *in* the _world_."
M. GANDHI

Change cannot happen until we take responsibility for our lives. Let's take care of ourselves even by cultivating something, getting our hands dirty, feeling useful in something with empathy.

We are the protagonists of our lives and by repeating positive actions we do nothing but lead us towards the desired result.

Set yourself achievable goals and start progressively but steadily to achieve them.

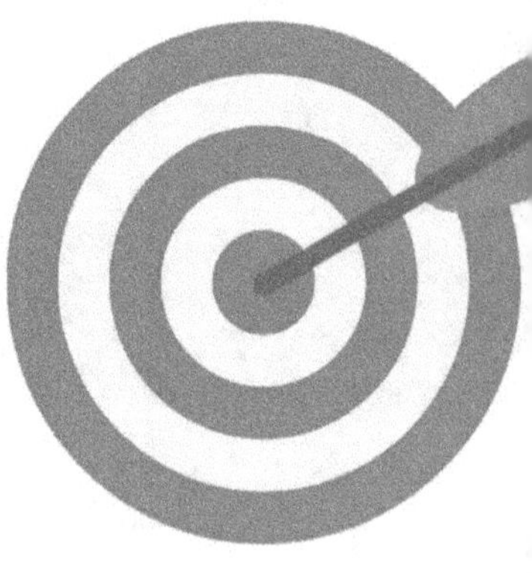

Always reward yourself in intermediate goals with your own pace.

Never give up!

"Never give up. It is usually the last key in the deck that opens the door."
PAULO COELHO

Among the readings I recommend I found very interesting *China study*, by Colin Campbell, and *La rivoluzione del glucosio* by Inchauspé and my book Forbidden to settle with Practical Coaching.

I wish you to find your well-being and your serenity.

"Good things come to those who believe, the best things come to those who *are patient, and extraordinary things come to those who don't give up.*"
ANONYMOUS

"*A winner is a dreamer who never gave up.*"
NELSON MANDELA

"I *can accept defeat, but I can't accept giving up trying.*"
MICHAEL JORDAN

The China Study

The most comprehensive nutrition study ever conducted

A monumental text with an important epidemiological study that lasted twenty-seven years and was carried out in collaboration with various universities. The American scientist T. Colin Campbell, together with his son Thomas M. Campbell II, analyze the relationship between diet and disease, coming to surprising conclusions. Finally, some of the fundamental theses that have always been supported by natural medicine are verified and tested: genetics is not the predominant factor in the genesis of diseases; Obsessive control of fats, carbohydrates, cholesterol and omega-3s does not result in good health; drugs and surgery do not cure the diseases we are suffering from; Doctors don't know exactly what to recommend to stay healthy; Only with diet and lifestyle can you recover from heart disease; Breast cancer is related to an altered hormonal situation that is determined by the food we eat; Dairy consumption increases the risk of prostate cancer; the antioxidants contained in fruits and vegetables are related to better mental performance in old age; Various types of cancer are related to excessive consumption of animal protein.

The glucose revolution: how to control blood sugar levels to lose weight, take away hunger and have more energy

Almost 90% of the population suffers from an excess of glucose in the blood, and most do not even know it.

The symptoms?

Hunger attacks, chronic fatigue, mood swings, skin problems, premature aging, infertility... and an increase, over time, in the risk of inflammatory diseases such as cardiovascular diseases, cancer, Alzheimer's and diabetes. With a rigorous scientific approach and an innovative method built over years of research, Jessie Inchauspé explains why glucose spikes are dangerous and how we can contain them without sacrificing the pleasure of food. Sweets and carbohydrates included.

It also explains how to lose weight effortlessly, how to store foods in the right order to lose weight without giving up your favorite dishes, what is the secret ingredient to enjoy a dessert without consequences, how to eatbreakfast in the morning to eliminate hunger attacks and turn fatigue into energy.

Biochemist Jessie Inchauspé analyzes the action of glucose on our body, finding the right nutritional solutions against the most common diseases.

The fastest and most effective way to lose weight, lower blood pressure and improve health involves flattening the glucose curve.

Just a few tricks related to nutrition r you can eat what you want!

1. Eat foods in the right order.

2. Always start with a green appetizer.

3. Stop counting calories.

4. Flatten the breakfast curve.

5. Choose any sugar, they are all the same.

6. Better a dessert than a snack.

7. A sip of vinegar before eating.

8. Move after eating.

9. Choose salty snacks.

10. Dress carbohydrates.

Ikigai for success: discover your talent and realize it

In the beginning was the Word, says the Gospel of John referring to the word that created us in the divine mind. In Japan this generative idea is called *ikigai* and indicates our original nature and the impulse that secretly drives all our actions. *Ikigai* is the note that distinguishes us from everyone and that makes us complementary to everyone, it is the seed from which the tree of our life is derived. In a historical period in which we have become credit card numbers, health cards, tax codes and computer passwords, rediscovering the value of our individual uniqueness is more important than ever, as is rediscovering the meaning of our life, the very reason why we exist, and thus combining personal happiness and professional fulfillment. The search for *ikigai* is therefore a real treasure hunt hidden in each of us and helps us to understand our added value compared to the world. An extraordinary discovery to which this book wants to guide us so that we can realize our deepest aspirations, finding our personal path to success and happiness.

Hanasaki: the Japanese art of living long and happy

From Japan come the nine principles to follow to be able to live peacefully and longer. Why is Japan the country with the longest life expectancy? Why are the Japanese among the people in the world who suffer the least from cancer and diabetes? The answer lies in nine fundamental pillars of Japanese living, which form the basis of the Hanasaki method. Like a "blooming flower", using some Japanese teachings, we can change, acquire a healthier lifestyle from a psychophysical point of view and even become better people.

What are these fundamental principles to take into account?

1. *Kaizen*: to obtain the tools that allow us to make lasting change. *Minimalism*: to focus on the essential and discard the superfluous.

2. *Inner peace*: to calm the movements of our spirit and live in harmony.

3. *Nature*: to reconnect with our origins.

4. *Health*: to transform us into strong and robust people.

5. *Relationships*: to establish deep and lasting bonds with others.

6. *Principles*: to find the light that illuminates our path.

7. *Ikigai*: to find meaning in our lives.

8. *Attitude*: to achieve what we propose and turn our dreams into reality.

A path that we should all walk.

Happiness : Your Guide for Self-Help,Self-

Esteem, Personal Growth, Stress

Management, using Practical Coaching

Exercises

& Mindfulness & Meditation

Here we go again! It's Monday and when the alarm goes off, thinking of going to the office or the day ahead you do not find the strength to get out of bed or even a real motivation to do so.

Maybe you don't like your job as much as you used to and try to remember when was the last time you woke up happy and **motivated**. You drag yourself forward and wondering if you could change company, or simply the job, or even start your own business by opening that business where you are so good and enjoy doing. And the days go by one after the other, equal to themselves, without you doing anything to change the situation. Then there is the crisis, the fear of the new and of **change**, or you have no idea where to start again.

In short, you are "**settling**".

Words are important. And often the meaning we give to a word is not the same for everyone. What is the difference between being content and accepting the situation?

- What is really important to us?
- What is my real talent?

These are questions that help us define what decision to make or focus on a goal.

Through many exercises, we will learn to take care of OURSELVES and improve our SELF-ESTEEM

Here are some exercises below.taken from my book.

Exercise with background music

Close your eyes, abandon yourself to chaos, trace on a sheet of paper a sign, the inspiration of the moment (your chaos). Now look at it, bring it to your mind, then get it out of your mind, make it dance in the air.

Every day imagine your drawing with your eyes closed.

What you want to achieve: activating the right hemisphere to stimulate creativity and make the left hemisphere outline the strategy to achieve the goals.

Each of us has a purpose in life already contained in our essence. To live means to achieve this goal by renouncing to please others.

Ask yourself: What world do I want to live in?

The answer is unconscious and will come at the right time.

Ask yourself: what can be my contribution to the world I desire? What do I leave to future generations?

Activation of the right hemisphere of the brain

Exercise 1: Search for your pet

Close your eyes, imagine that you are an animal, feel like an animal in your breath, in your posture. What animal are you? What are your qualities? What do you want for yourself and the world?

<u>*Exercise 2: Rewrite your story*</u>

If you had three lives, what would you do? Who would you be? What would your day be like? Write on the fly. Choose one of these lives and write down who you are, what you really want.

Exercise 3: Your outlook on life

What do you want for your life?

What do you want for the world?

What are the qualities only yours?

Choose the most important ones and you will find your vision of life. Then close your eyes, imagine yourself in a few years. Who are you with?

Where are you?

How do you also feel physically with your vision?

Make yourself like you're creating a positive situation for yourself. Then imagine speaking from the future, from that time and place.

What positive effect will you have on others?

What resources will you use?

What critical moments will you encounter and how will you resolve them?

Observe yourself: seeing yourself from the future, what advice would you give yourself?

Have you wondered if you are living the life you wanted and if you are proud of it?

What are the five things you're proud of?

What do you want to accomplish in life to feel that you have lived fully?

How many times has fear blocked you, preventing you from reaching your goal?

Ask yourself now what you want.

Focus now only on what you are doing. Write or record your voice as you talk about the goals you have in mind to store positive, repeatable thoughts over multiple days.

Daniel Goleman groups stress into anger, anxiety and sorrow that sadden all existence. Anxiety takes away energy well-being, obstacles seem insurmountable to you, and you feel sad and frustrated.

Why not engage in creativity? Enter a list of calming activities here, such as listening to classical music, so you know that happiness is always with us.

Negative thoughts often overwhelm us in the form of this inner voice that accompanies us, the voice of yesterday's mistakes and our fears that exhausts us and makes us devoid of energy.

Are you afraid of being judged by your loved ones? Are you looking for perfection?

"I thought too much," the mentor explained, "I was mulling over, but without the help of the psychologist I changed my lifestyle, I learned to accept myself as I am, I did a lot of exercise, I set achievable goals."

Now ask yourself: is this thought useful for me? How does it make me feel?

Write a journal or record your voice and write down the ten good things you did in a day. If you feel disoriented, unmotivated, ask yourself how you will feel in six months?

How will your health be with a new lifestyle, doing sports three times a week?

I recommend, reward yourself when you reach the intermediate results.

A new way of being

with mindfulness

The practice of mindfulness sees as its main objective the achievement of a maximum degree of awareness through which the individual should reach a state of well-being. By becoming aware and not critical of themselves and reality, individuals should be able to control and contain negative emotions, sensations, and thoughts that can lead to suffering.

What mindfulness is NOT:

- It is NOT a mystical experience;
- It is NOT a way to escape the problems of reality: on the contrary, mindfulness is practiced to understand and analyze it in the present moment and in a non-judgmental way;
- It is NOT psychotherapy.

One way to cultivate *mindfulness* in everyday life is to eat slowly, sitting at the table, and without distractions. Focusing only on the act of eating, pay attention to the aromas, savor every bite, pay attention to how you cut food, how you feel while eating.

Do you feel pleasure? What experience did it give you on a sensory level? If you behaved like this in everything you do, what would your life be like?

This is a method to manage Nervous Hunger.

Emotional hunger comes precisely in moments of weakness. It comes in those cases in which our mind alone can not manage situations of stress or depression and, the only easiest and most pleasant way, finds it in food and to lift the mood we dive into fatty or sweet foods, which somehow give gratification.

And mindfulness allows you to tune into your physical signals of natural hunger.

Eating "Mindful" means transforming an often hurried and superficial moment into an opportunity for contact with oneself. It is necessary to dedicate a precise time to "eating", avoiding polluting the time of the meal with other activities such as working on the computer.

Now let's talk about thoughts. Pay attention to how your mind swells and deflates with thoughts, try to observe them as an external subject, without being clinging to them, without rejecting them, considering them as objects that appear and disappear. Can you observe them? Otherwise you can always anchor yourself to the breath and focus on it.

Desiring the good and joy for oneself and for others allows one to better manage difficult emotions. According to *mindfulness*, intentions are formulated by repeating four phrases addressed to yourself, to a dear friend, to a difficult person, to a person who is neutral for you and to the whole world like:

- "May we... be happy."
- "May we... be safe."
- "May we... be healthy."
- "May we... live in peace."

This is the procedure for being kind and loving towards ourselves and others and will have to be repeated throughout the day.

Thanks to the mental clarity that *mindfulness* teaches you , you will become aware of this flow of thoughts, from acceptance to fear, understanding how futile we are looking for changing thoughts and being at the mercy of them. With loving-kindness you will relax, without opposing thoughts, honoring yourself and committing yourself to others, spreading happiness in the world. The change often mentioned in this manual is constant and illusory in our thoughts.

Surrendering to the flow of life will bring you closer to the real you, achieving the sense of fullness and true purpose of your existence. You will not compare yourself to others, you will ask yourself what you have to defend in the world?

Lucia is a woman who has work as her primary value, has a strong sense of duty and tends to criticize herself. The concept of flexibility was not envisaged by you. If a colleague wasted time, they would immediately take action to fix the problem. She was obsessed with perfection, so much so that she never felt up to any situation, until she discovered *mindfulness* and the positive aspect of letting go.

Here are some examples of *mindfulness-based* breathing.

Exercise

Place one hand on your chest and the other on your belly. In your mind's eye, imagine that behind your navel is a balloon that gradually fills with air as you inhale and empties when you exhale. Make your belly relax.

Let your breath guide you, trying to feel its rhythm. With time the breathing will slow down and become deeper to the natural rhythm.

Stretch your arms along your sides imagining you are on a mattress in the middle of the sea, when you inhale the belly swells slowly, when you exhale the belly deflates slowly.

How are you feeling?

Once you have finished observing yourself, you can open your eyes.

Gratitude mindfulness exercise

Now you can perform another meditation. Find a comfortable position and close your eyes.

Notice that each breath is different, exhale and say, "I am grateful." Feel the feeling of gratitude for life.

Inhale and exhale, saying, "I am calm." Let the tranquility expand in you.

Inhale and exhale and slumber all sensations throughout the day.

Mindfulness for self-esteem

This is the journey to self-esteem, acceptance and loving-kindness. Anchor yourself in your breath and turn to the present moment.

Meditation is an important pillar as it leads to inner peace. Have you ever tried this practice?

The positive effect will make you satisfied and make you realize that improving is an easy process.

Meditation only works if you take the time and find the right place to experience it.

Once you have gained some practice, you will begin to use positive words to bring out the inner balance you need. Not everything will always go according to plan, if you feel an improvement, you will be ready to move on.

Learn the *Mindfulness* of Breathing

This *mindfulness* technique consists of detaching oneself from one's thoughts and emotions, seeing them as an external observer. As you observe your thoughts, work to recognize and define negativity.

Practice *mindfulness* to resist urgencies, impulses, and pressing desires.

Mindfulness involves a form of meditation in which we observe our feelings without judging them.

A technique to combat stress for a tired mind

How to fight stress and stay calm? Soak in a hot tub to relieve muscle aches. It works wonders even for a tired mind.

If you do not know how to meditate, try listening to a podcast, there are several that can guide you step by step. Music is also a great way to relax and improve your mood. Surround yourself with positive people who exert a calming influence; Don't spend time with people who belittle you. Learn to say no, take control of the parts of your life that you can change, that cause you stress. Being selective about what you face and saying no to things that will unnecessarily add to your load are two actions that can reduce stress levels.

Consider that there are supplements to reduce stress and anxiety such as lemon balm, valerian, also reduce exciting foods such as tea, coffee, chocolate and spend more time with friends.

Eliminate anxious thoughts from your head, writing them in a journal, recording them. Write down all your concerns, also be grateful and focus on the positive thoughts in your life. At the end of the day you can replace rational thoughts with more useful and positive ones, writing can help you get to know yourself better. Sleep the right time, use supplements, such as melatonin, which will replenish energy levels and concentration.

Lucia embarked on this journey with great confidence and learned to let go and not always be obsessed with perfection and felt less and less stressed.

Anna Laura, successful entrepreneur, focused on a fast career, is very practical and attentive to the dress, moves with a decisive step and is a woman who makes noise in the corridor just walking. Anna Laura wants others to notice her. However, she complained that she did not have time to be with her children and writing down the positive and negative characteristics of her parents made her aware that stress at work made her lose the energy destined for her family. Having started to dedicate herself to herself has changed her life and also her employment.

Gaia is a thinker, she is very wise but she lives isolated from the world. She reads many books and is always passionate about new things, she fears not being able to achieve her goals and the dormant anger consumes her and makes her stay away from others. Thanks to meditation she was able to recover, to look inside and find her life, to resume her true passion, painting.

Exercise to anchor states of trust in our ego
Imitate in a shopping mall a person who seems self-confident, his posture, his stride...

How do you feel inside? How can we create constructive sensations? How can we anchor states of trust?

Exercise to improve our self-esteem

This method will help you to make the fear disappear for an interview, to deal with a difficult colleague and in many other situations.

Cut out a circle with paper and color it orange, then cut out a square and color it blue.

Put the square on the floor.

Think of a situation where you were unsure of yourself. Notice the sensations.

Get out of the paper and think about how you'll feel the next time that happens.

Now remember a beautiful experience in which you were confident.

Place the orange circle, which symbolizes energy, and with your eyes turned upwards remember the situation, magnify it with your imagination, let all the sensations you perceive flow. Bring the image closer and closer. Enjoy the well-being and smile. Look at the blue square and how you have changed. Pick up the circle and return to the square. Imagine the old situation with renewed confidence.
Positive emotions improve skills.

Your Soul is a unique treasure chest that needs deep growth, you need to accept the past and change your life. Your change is your new well-being and you will know how to reassure yourself in your Path of Life.
Good life
Coach Lola

About the author

Lola Steven is a Certified Coach and also specializes in Mindfulness.

The practices of compassion, mindfulness, and loving-kindness helped her face her difficulties and grow through her young adulthood. Her passion lies in investigating the ancient teachings, and how they are relevant to our modern life.

Recommended Books

https://www.amazon.com/Powerful-Mind-YOURSELF-overthinking-Personal-ebook/dp/B0CGRN2927/ref=sr_1_1?crid=546NXYZ74JRG&keywords=lola+steven&qid=1697698453&sprefix=lola+steven%2Caps%2C190&sr=8-1

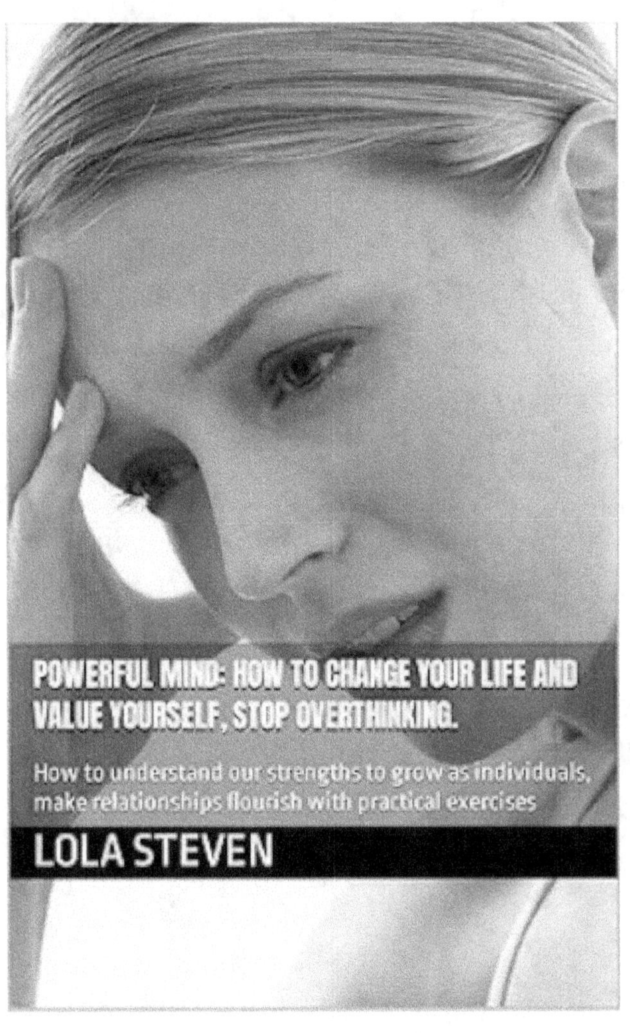

Overthinking is the biggest cause of unhappiness. Don't get stuck in a never-ending thought loop. Stay present and keep your mind off things that don't matter, and never   will.

Stop Overthinking is a book that understands where you've been through,the exhausting situation you've put yourself into, and how you lose your mind in the trap of anxiety and stress.

Stop agonizing over the past and trying to predict the future.

Powerful ways to stop ruminating and dwelling on negative thoughts.

https://www.amazon.com/STRATEGIES-BE-HAPPIER-POSITIVE-THOUGHTS-ebook/dp/B0C9HYPR6T/ref=sr_1_2?crid=546NXYZ74JRG&keywords=lola+steven&qid=169

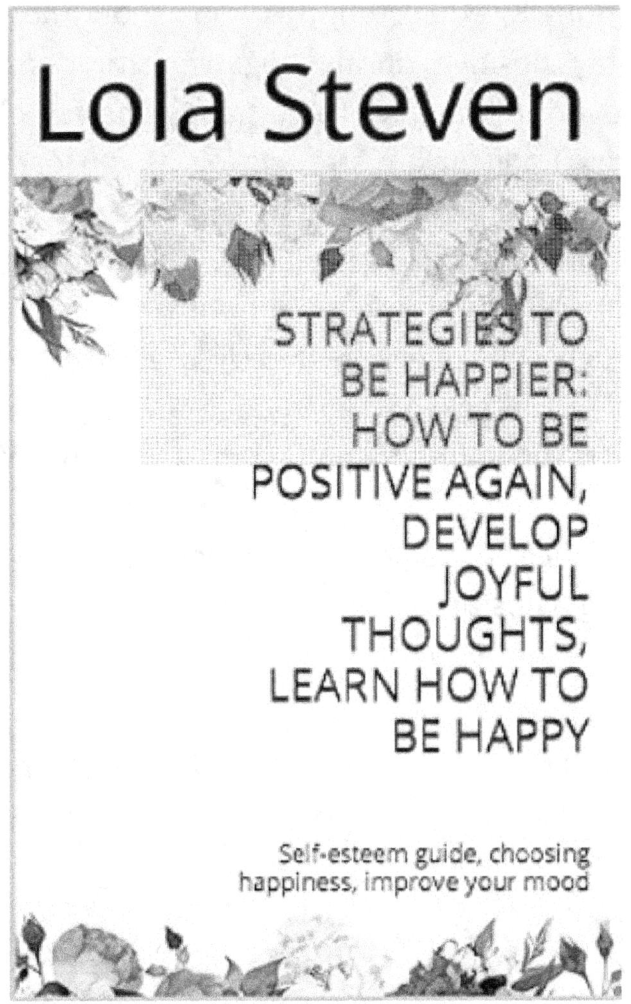
Lola Steven
STRATEGIES TO
BE HAPPIER:
HOW TO BE
POSITIVE AGAIN,
DEVELOP
JOYFUL
THOUGHTS,
LEARN HOW TO
BE HAPPY
Self-esteem guide, choosing
happiness, improve your mood

Stop wanting to be more positive and just do it! For anyone who is tired of feeling emotionally exhausted, this book shows how to stay positive during negative situations. Discover all the ways to be happy and full of energy. Reduce your stress levels as you learn to stay calm during times of negativity. Find your power of positivity. Look for the bright side and move on with your life. Through self-reflection exercises at the end of the chapter, you can reduce the negative aspects of your life and start a life full of more   positivity. Experience a healthier, happier you while getting a positive outlook.

https://www.amazon.com/Happiness-Self-Esteem-Management-Mindfulness-Meditation-ebook/dp/B0C4Y4NX95/ref=sr_1_3?crid=546NXYZ74JRG&keywords=lola+steven&qid=169

7698511&sprefix=lola+steven%2Caps%2C190
&sr=8-3

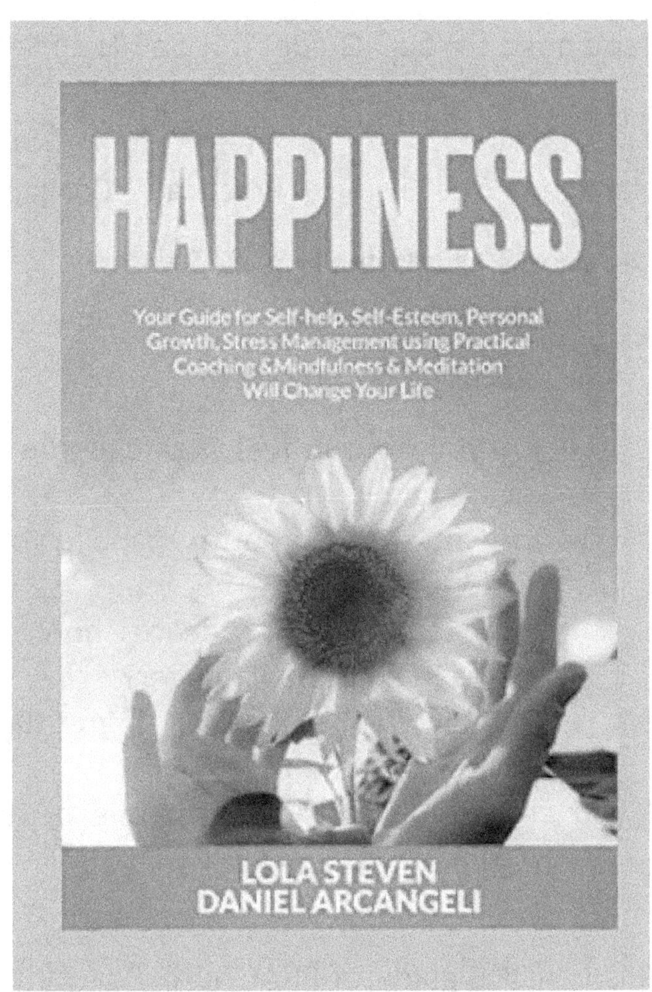

HAPPINESS
Your Guide for Self-help, Self-Esteem, Personal Growth, Stress Management using Practical Coaching & Mindfulness & Meditation Will Change Your Life
LOLA STEVEN
DANIEL ARCANGELI

Happiness : Your Guide for Self-Help, Self-Esteem, Personal Growth, Stress Management, using Practical Coaching Exercises & Mindfulness & Meditation

- **Want to be happier?**

- Do you want to feel as safe as you've ever been?
- Do you want to better manage your children?
- Do you want to learn how to manage emotional hunger?
- Do you want to feel full of gratitude in every situation?

If you answered yes to at least one of the questions, then this is the book for you!

This UNIQUE guide of PRACTICAL Coaching is for all people who truly want to have more power and more happiness in their lives thus creating their own destiny.

Practical Coaching: Discover Your Potential Improve Your Self-esteem & Unleash Your Talent & Improve Your Relationships", a self-help manual written, through reflection points and exercises to eliminate new limiting beliefs and will gently transport you towards the flowering of a new awareness, to find the strength and enthusiasm to live life feeling in harmony with yourself, with others and with the whole universe.

You have always been told that to be happy you need to improve and change, but it is a wrong and useless effort.
We must learn to listen to ourselves and let our uniqueness emerge, the only source of true happiness.
Here is the way to be yourself: free yourself from models and roles, from managing our life and also our nutrition, learning to observe without judging, opening your mind to the new and the unexpected

https://www.amazon.com/ALWAYS-STAY-YOUNG-Centenarians-Personal-ebook/dp/B0CGDWGGRV/ref=sr_1_4?crid=5 46NXYZ74JRG&keywords=lola+steven&qid=1 697698511&sprefix=lola+steven%2Caps%2C1 90&sr=8-4

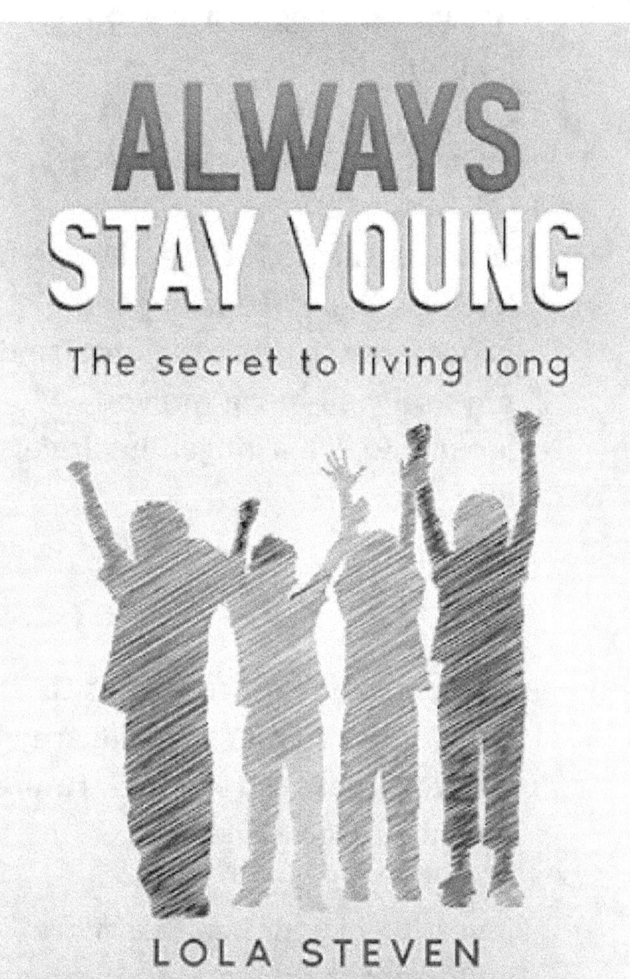

ALWAYS
STAY YOUNG
The secret to living long
LOLA STEVEN

Are you seeking to live a longer, healthier life?

If so, you're in the right place.

Discover the secret to achieving lasting vitality, from longer life expectancy to greater mental and physical well-being Are you looking to live a longer, healthier life?

If so, you're not alone...

As life expectancy continues to rise, more and more people are realizing that securing their future means planning ahead.

Investing in your health is more important than ever, but it can be difficult to know what you need to do to optimize your functioning in the future.

You may have heard that diet and exercise are essential to living a long and healthy life.

While this is true, there is much more to living well with age.

Your well-being isn't just defined by your diet and exercise habits. The strength of your relationships, the positive vibes you cultivate in your mindset.

In fact, research shows that how you plan to age can influence what happens.

This guide offers an innovative approach to health by addressing physical, mental and emotional well-being in one place.

Packed with inspiring evidence for a holistic lifestyle, it provides the tools you need to bring lasting transformation into your daily life.

Arm yourself with the knowledge you need to live a longer, healthier life, no matter where you currently are.

With the right roadmap, you can chart a different path for your life, one that allows you to survive your genes to make each decade better than the previous one.

If you are ready to become the architect of your own health and unlock a life of well-being, scroll up and click the "Add to Cart" button right now.

In this guide you'll discover :

AGEING..
SLOWING DOWN AGING: THE
SECRETS TO STAYING YOUNG AND
HEALTHY.

Free radicals.

Antioxidants: friends for the skin.

Healthy habits to stay young
longer.

A MEANINGFUL LIFE HELPS TO
LIVE LONG.

ACCEPT WHAT WE ARE

THE IMPORTANCE OF GLUCOSE

THE BENEFITS OF EXERCISE

Pilates Method

The 8 fundamental principles of the Pilates Method.

A HINT OF EMOTIONAL HEALING: NEGATIVE ION THERAPY.

Getting older shouldn't be a daunting experience – they're called the golden years for a reason!

Don't spend another day stuck in old routines and habits holding you back.

If you are ready to become the ruler of your health and your wellness, then scroll up and click the "Add to Cart" button right now.

https://www.amazon.com/gp/product/B0CD
875M98?ref_=dbs_m_mng_rwt_calw_tkin_2
&storeType=ebooks&qid=1697699702&sr=1-
11

https://www.amazon.com/FELICITA-
EMOTIVA-CRESCITA-PERSONALE-Personale-
ebook/dp/B0C2TNV9NC/ref=sr_1_1?crid=VU
YXDQ0FDKS8&keywords=daniela+arcangeli&
qid=1697698185&sprefix=daniela+arcangeli%
2Caps%2C178&sr=8-1

FELICITA' EMOTIVA : GUIDA PER UNA VITA FELICE per la CRESCITA PERSONALE con Bambino interiore, con i Chakra, fiori australiani, cure con ioni ... alla Crescita Personale) (Italian Edition)

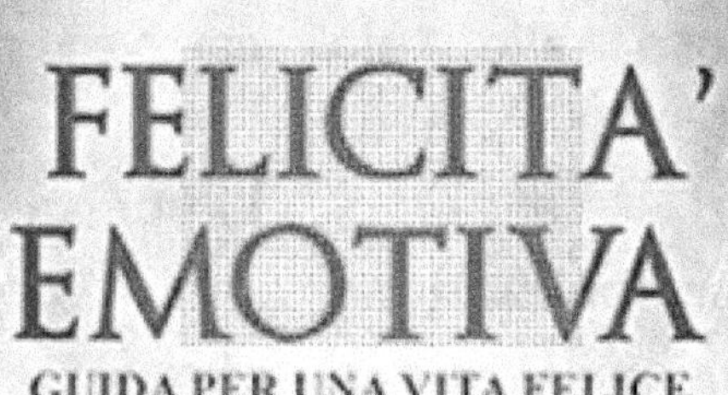

FELICITA'
EMOTIVA
GUIDA PER UNA VITA FELICE
per la CRESCITA PERSONALE
Come smettere di pensare troppo, imparare ad essere sereni
e ad avere pensieri positivi e come gestire i pensieri negativi
DANIELA ARCANGELI

Le emozioni stanno alla base di tutte le nostre azioni, dalle più virtuose alle più cattive per l'AUTOSTIMA.

Scopri l'importanza dell'armonizzazione della guarigione energetica ed emozionale per il raggiungimento del benessere psico-fisico e l'autoguarigione per il raggiungimento della felicità.

Come smettere di pensare troppo, imparare ad essere sereni e ad avere pensieri positivi e come gestire i pensieri negativi

**Senti il bisogno di un rimuginio continuo con senso di pesantezza e stanchezza?
Hai la sensazione di rincorrere la stabilità senza raggiungerla?
O semplicemente stai iniziando il tuo percorso di crescita personale con lo scopo di riuscire finalmente a vedere la vita per quello che è realmente?**

L'autrice, Daniela Arcangeli è una Coach certificata da International Coaching Federation e Naturopata che utilizza molti metodi di guarigione emozionale e metodi per migliorare l'AUTOSTIMA.

Stress, irrequietezza e instabilità sono le conseguenze più diffuse di questi tempi frenetici e spesso proprio loro ti conducono a sentirti demotivato. Imparare che non puoi riuscire a controllare la vita rappresenta il primo passo per tornare a percorrerla attraverso una sana accettazione degli eventi. In questo processo avrai a disposizione molteplici metodi che ti permetteranno di affrontare al meglio il tuo cammino di crescita personale verso la rinascita.

Attraverso i CHAKRA, il coaching, i fiori australiani, le COSTELLAZIONI FAMILIARI comprenderai meglio te stesso in ogni tuo aspetto. Solo comprendendo le piccole cose infatti e l'importanza che hanno nel grande disegno della vita verso l'elevazione spirituale, potrai ritrovare te stesso e ritornare ad essere felice.

Grazie a questo libro potrai conoscere e comprendere la funzione delle varie tecniche in un percorso guidato che ti permetterà inoltre di:

- Riequilibrare la tua energia emozionale attraverso il tuo bambino interiore e migliorare l'AUTOSTIMA;
- Imparare un metodo per armonizzare i tuoi Chakra;
- 3 meditazioni di guarigione;
- I fiori di bach e i fiori australiani:

- <u>La ionoterapia per riequilibrare la tua energia;</u>
- <u>Il coaching e le costellazioni familiari</u>
-

Ogni esperienza proposta viene spiegata in modo dettagliato per permettere anche ai principianti di effettuare le pratiche e trovare quella più adatta a loro.

<u>Con l'acquisto di questo libro sarà inoltre possibile scaricare 3 meditazioni audio guidate</u> per la tua guarigione

Riprendi il potere della tua vita mettendoti finalmente al primo posto, sii FELICE, scorri verso l'alto e clicca su "Acquista ora"!

Ecco un brano del libro

È importante consolare il tuo bambino interiore.

Ecco un metodo espresso in modo metaforico che trovate nel mio libro _Noi piccoli uomini saggi_. La protagonista è Adele, che vuole entrare in contatto con la sua bambina interiore.

«_Come posso, ora, entrare in contatto con lei che forse non vorrà più dialogare con me?_

Me la immagino rinchiusa in un vecchio baule, sommersa da mille e più cianfrusaglie: per un po' di tempo ha cercato di farsi largo tra i pesi che la opprimevano, ma quando ha capito che ero forte, o meglio che cercavo di sembrarlo, ha rinunciato. Si è dibattuta, ma ha ceduto. Può veramente emergere dal fondo del baule?» concluse con voce tremante.

«Fai le cose con calma e prenditi tutto il tempo che ti è necessario. Prova a dirle che le vuoi bene. Immagina di prenderla per mano e di trascorrere con lei qualche giorno felice.

Adulto e bambina dovranno comunicarsi ogni cosa e qualsiasi cosa accada, l'adulto non scapperà, sarà sempre disponibile.»

«È proprio necessario farlo? Non so se sono pronta» disse Adele.

«Ti sei dimenticata di lei per quarant'anni e ci potrà volere tempo prima che risponda. Rilassati e chiudi gli occhi… Dille che vuoi parlarle, che vuoi vederla, amarla…»

Adele si rilassò. Chiese alla bambina di poterle parlare, insistette per un po' di volte. ma alla fine questa apparve di fronte a lei. Era forse triste, mentre canticchiava qualcosa a bassa voce, indossava un vestitino rosa, ornato di tanti fiocchi, e sulle spalle lunghi capelli ricci. Adele aveva le lacrime agli occhi: aveva appoggiato il mento sulla sua stessa mano e la guardava.

Deglutì per non mettersi a piangere, le chiese perdono per essersi dimenticata di lei per così tanto tempo e poi, con voce tremula, espresse la domanda che le aveva suggerito il libro:

«Che cosa ti spaventa ancora?»

La bambina rispose che trovava enormi difficoltà nell'affezionarsi completamente a qualcuno.

«Che cosa posso fare per evitarti tutto questo?» chiese la donna.

La bambina aveva in mano una bambola e, mentre le spazzolava la lucente chioma, la guardava e sorrideva intimidita meravigliandosi per quello che vedeva. All'improvviso, sbattendo gli occhioni, disse: «Fammi giocare... ho voglia di divertirmi, come nei momenti più belli in cui ero con papà».

Adele rimase perplessa da questa richiesta, ma il libro intervenne.

«Trova un po' di tempo per te, Adele, non ti preoccupare, non avere timori e chiedi alla bambina che cosa le piacerebbe nello specifico. Se lei ti risponde ancora, vuol dire che sei entrata finalmente in comunicazione con te stessa...»

Adele prese il coraggio: ci voleva una grande forza d'animo per parlare così a se stessa.

Adele chiese alla bambina se voleva disegnare, come faceva una volta. La bambina spalancò gli occhi e gridò il suo sì, entusiasta.

Il libro intervenne a questo punto per spiegare meglio cosa si poteva fare con il disegno.

«Adele, prendi i pennarelli o dei pastelli e, usando la mano non dominante, disegnati da bambina. Cerca di comprendere che cosa ti suggerisce il disegno, considera i colori che hai usato e che cosa stai facendo...»

Adele disegnò se stessa con un grande sorriso, in una specie di inchino, e accanto a sé disegnò una casetta con il fumo che usciva dal tetto. I colori che aveva usato erano il verde, il rosso, il giallo.

https://www.amazon.com/Vietato-accontentarsi-Coaching-Pratico-rimandando-ebook/dp/B0C7QMHYN1/ref=sr_1_2?crid=VUYXDQ0FDKS8&keywords=daniela+arcangeli&qid=1697698198&sprefix=daniela+arcangeli%2Caps%2C178&sr=8-2

Vietato accontentarsi con il Coaching Pratico: Stai rimandando una decisione, ti arrovelli pensando a come uscire da una situazione un po' scomoda

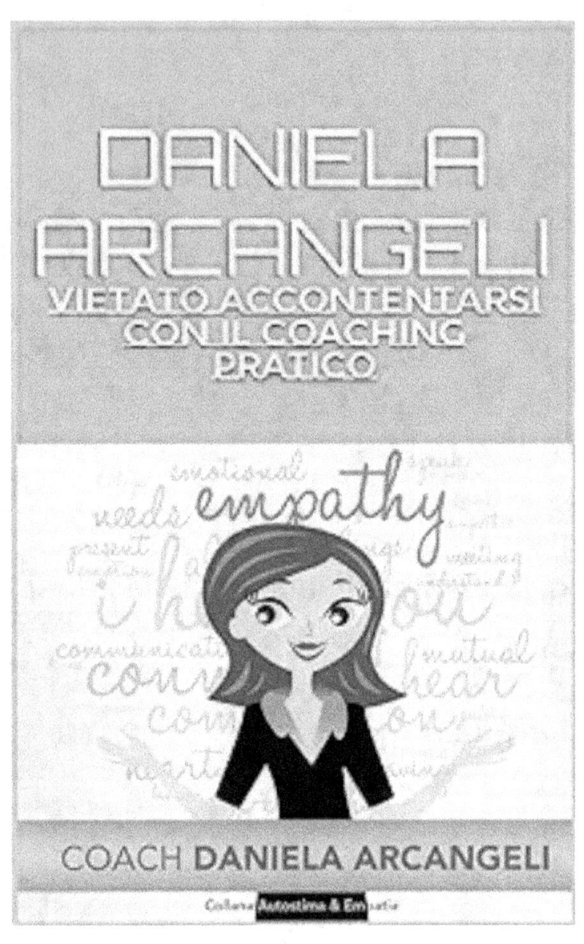

DANIELA ARCANGELI
VIETATO ACCONTENTARSI
CON IL COACHING
PRATICO
empathy
COACH DANIELA ARCANGELI

Ecco, ci risiamo! è lunedì e quando suona la sveglia, pensando di andare in ufficio o alla giornata che ti aspetta non trovi la forza di alzarti dal letto e neanche una vera motivazione per farlo.

Magari il tuo lavoro non ti piace più come una volta e cerchi di ricordare quando è stata l'ultima volta che ti sei svegliato felice e motivato. Ti trascini andando avanti e chiedendoti se potresti cambiare azienda, o semplicemente la mansione, o addirittura metterti in proprio aprendo quell'attività in cui sei tanto bravo e ti diverti a fare. E i giorni passano uno dopo l'altro, uguali a se stessi, senza che tu faccia qualcosa per cambiare la situazione. Poi c'è la crisi, la paura del nuovo e del cambiamento, o non hai idea da dove ripartire.

In poche parole ti stai "accontentando".

Le parole sono importanti. E spesso il significato che diamo ad una parola non è uguale per tutti.

Che differenza c'è tra accontentarsi e accettare la situazione?

- Cosa è davvero importante per noi?

- Qual è un mio vero talento?

Queste sono domande che ci aiutano a definire quale decisione prendere o focalizzare un obiettivo Attraverso tantissimi esercizi, impareremo ad avere cura di NOI STESSI e a migliorare la nostra AUTOSTIMA

Ecco un estratto del libro

In questo capitolo ti si presenterà un'altra opportunità da cogliere.

Prendiamo l'esempio di Armando, che si sentiva soddisfatto della sua vita lavorativa e non capiva quale malessere poteva avere dentro, anche se un campanellino si azionava in certi momenti della giornata. Tutti lo vedevano arrivato, aveva una bella famiglia, era una persona di successo, pareva che non avesse bisogno di altro. Non è difficile per un top manager ammettere che qualcosa non va, è difficile capire i propri bisogni, i propri valori e i danni che si fanno non osservandoli in profondità. Ritornare a essere felici non è facile, soprattutto azzerando il passato, ma lui lo fece.

Il cambiamento è la vita, il fine è diventare consapevoli e il nostro obiettivo è la felicità, il modo non è univoco, l'obiettivo è l'evoluzione e il ritrovamento di se stessi. La cosa peggiore non è fallire, è non provarci. Il dolore non si può evitare, fa parte della vita, puoi "solo" influenzare il modo di vivere gli eventi.

Ti sei domandato se stai vivendo la vita che volevi e se ne sei orgoglioso?

Queste furono le prime domande che si fece Armando.

Armando si ispirò al suo mentore di sempre, il suo professore di filosofia. Lo aveva sempre ammirato quando andava a scuola.

Le sue domande lo avevano ogni volta coinvolto o sconvolto e dopo tanti anni di distanza dalla scuola, gli rimanevano dentro nell'anima.

Quali sono le cinque cose di cui vai fiero?

Cosa vuoi realizzare nella vita per sentire che hai vissuto appieno?

Quante volte la paura ti ha bloccato, impedendoti di raggiungere l'obiettivo?

«La paura è il tuo dialogo interiore, la voce che potenzialmente ti fa ricordare tutti i fallimenti, se la stessa voce ci incitasse, ci rendesse vincenti, cambierebbero i nostri risultati» gli diceva sempre a lezione.

Domandati ora cosa vuoi.

Concentrati ora solo su quello che stai facendo. Scrivi o registra la tua voce mentre parli degli obiettivi che hai in mente per immagazzinare pensieri positivi e ripetibili per più giorni.

RESTARE SEMPRE GIOVANI: Come rimanere giovani dentro, fuori e nella mente

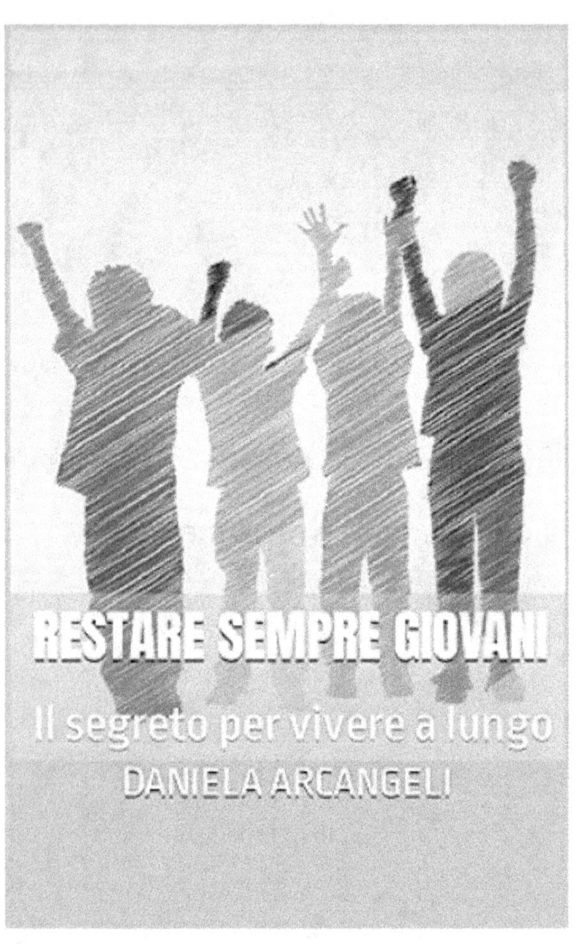

RESTARE SEMPRE GIOVANI
Il segreto per vivere a lungo
DANIELA ARCANGELI

Scopri il segreto per raggiungere una vitalità duratura, da una maggiore aspettativa di vita a un maggiore benessere mentale e fisico
Stai cercando di vivere una vita più lunga e più sana?

Se è così, non sei solo...

Mentre l'aspettativa di vita continua ad aumentare, sempre più persone si stanno rendendo conto del fatto che garantire il proprio futuro significa pianificare in anticipo.

Investire nella tua salute è più importante che mai, ma può essere difficile sapere cosa devi fare per ottimizzare il funzionamento in futuro.

Potresti aver sentito che la dieta e l'esercizio fisico sono essenziali per vivere una vita lunga e salutare.

Mentre questo è vero, c'è molto di più di questi due aspetti per vivere bene con l'età.

Il tuo benessere non è solo definito dalla tua dieta e dalle tue abitudini di esercizio. La forza delle tue relazioni, le vibrazioni positive che coltivi nella tua mentalità.

In effetti, la ricerca mostra che il modo in cui prevedi di invecchiare può influenzare ciò che accade.

Questa guida offre un approccio innovativo alla salute affrontando il benessere fisico, mentale ed emotivo in un unico posto.

Ricco di prove stimolanti per uno stile di vita olistico, fornisce gli strumenti necessari per portare una trasformazione duratura nella tua vita quotidiana.

Armati delle conoscenze di cui hai bisogno per vivere una vita più lunga e più sana, indipendentemente da dove ti trovi attualmente.

Con la giusta tabella di marcia, puoi tracciare un percorso diverso per la tua vita, uno che ti permetta di sopravvivere ai tuoi geni per rendere ogni decennio migliore di quello precedente.

Se sei pronto a diventare l'artefice della tua salute e sbloccare una vita di benessere, scorri verso l'alto e fai clic sul pulsante

"Aggiungi al carrello" in questo momento.

L'invecchiamento è stato a lungo considerato un processo normale. Pensiamo che la malattia, la fragilità e il declino graduale siano parti inevitabili della vita. Ma non devono esserlo. La scienza oggi vede l'invecchiamento come una malattia curabile. Affrontando le sue cause alla radice non solo possiamo aumentare la nostra durata della salute e vivere più a lungo, ma prevenire e invertire le malattie dell'invecchiamento, tra cui malattie cardiache, cancro, diabete

Ecco un brano del libro

Quello che motiva tutti i giorni le persone è vivere secondo la propria *mission*. Questa è una domanda che mi sono sempre posta, perché sono al mondo? Qual è il mio ruolo nel mondo?

Mi sono capitati tra le mani alcuni libri sull'*ikigai* e ho voluto condividerli con te. Il mio *ikigai* è aiutare a migliorare, direi che ci siamo, in ogni momento da quando mi sono laureata, il mio obiettivo è stato questo e lo confermo, in ogni società, in ogni situazione e quando non l'ho fatto, i risultati sono stati pessimi.

La filosofia dell'*ikigai* ha origine nell'antico Giappone nel 794 e si sviluppa fino al 1185. Trova la sua diffusione nel 1966 grazie alla pubblicazione del libro *ikigai* sul senso della vita dello psichiatra giapponese Kamiya.

Akihiro Asegawa, psicologo clinico, introdusse nel 2001 l'*ikigai* nella lingua giapponese E si scoprì più tardi che esso era uno dei segreti della straordinaria longevità della popolazione dell'isola di Okinawa.

Conoscere lo scopo della propria vita e il valore della propria unicità è l'inizio della nostra guarigione emozionale e della nostra salute psicofisica.

Per trovare l'*ikigai* è necessario sottoporsi a un test attitudinale e quando individuiamo in modo preciso il nostro *ikigai* esso è per sempre. Il senso della nostra vita è trovare il nostro dono per donarlo agli altri. Nel momento in cui troviamo il nostro *ikigai* ciascuno può riconoscere se stesso nella sua essenza più vera. L'*ikigai* è usato come un efficace metodo di selezione e di formazione del personale per costruire squadre di lavoro motivate ed efficienti.

Cosa cambia nella nostra vita quando troviamo l'*ikigai*? Cambia tutto perché da quel momento capiamo che cosa è davvero essenziale per noi e smettiamo di essere inutile a noi stessi trasformandoci in un vero e proprio dono.

Le domande sono 56 e di seguito vi propongo alcune delle domande che possono essere importanti per ottenere il vostro *ikigai*:

- di cosa mi appassiona parlare a lungo con i miei amici? Dai almeno tre risposte.

- Ho un'intera giornata libera, come mi piacerebbe trascorrerla? Dai almeno tre risposte.

- Quali sono le cose le persone o le circostanze che mi caricano di energia? Dai almeno tre risposte.

- Quali sono le cose che faccio con maggior piacere? Dai almeno tre risposte.

- Per quali qualità ricevo più spesso complimenti o elogi? Dai almeno tre risposte.

- Che cosa sono disposto a fare anche gratis solo per il piacere di farlo? Dai almeno tre risposte

- Di cosa hanno più bisogno il mondo e l'umanità? Dai almeno cinque risposte.

ESERCIZI QUOTIDIANI DI CREATIVITA' ANTI STRESS:COLTIVA LA TUA IMMAGINAZIONE LA

TUA ISPIRAZIONE: Sblocca il tuo potenziale creativo e vivi una VITA appagante

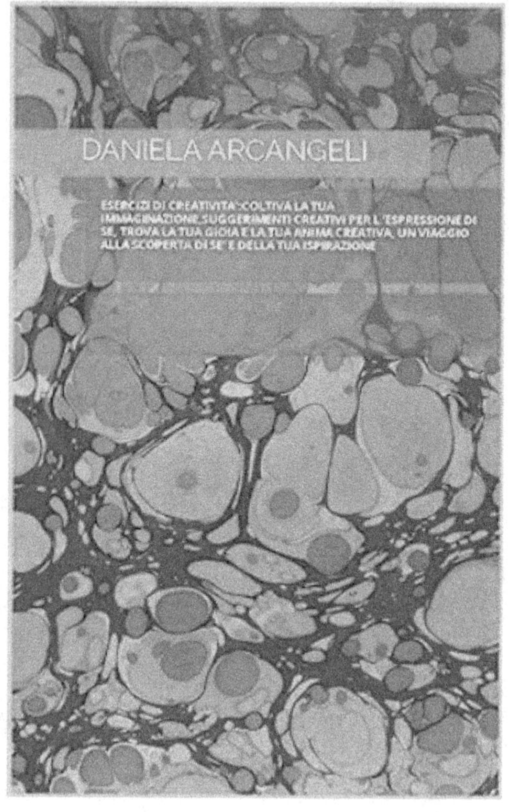

Il libro va ben oltre fornendo esercizi e approfondimenti attuabili, rendendo facile applicare i concetti nella vita reale. Ciò che distingue questa guida è la sua semplicità e accessibilità. Non è necessario essere esperti di psicologia o creatività per comprendere e beneficiare della saggezza all'interno di queste pagine.

Uno dei punti chiave di questo libro è l'idea di vivere nel momento presente. Ci ricorda che non possiamo cambiare il passato, ma possiamo plasmare il nostro futuro attraverso una vita consapevole e un pensiero positivo. La promessa di trovare la pace mentale e sbloccare il tuo potenziale creativo è a portata di clic.

Non lasciare che i pensieri negativi

controllino più la tua vita. Prendi in mano il tuo destino oggi stesso afferrando una copia di questo libro. È un piccolo investimento con il potenziale di produrre risultati che cambiano la vita. Sono grato per aver scoperto questa guida e sono fiducioso che porterà cambiamenti positivi anche alla tua vita. Dì addio all'essere schiavo dei tuoi pensieri e intraprendi un viaggio di auto-scoperta e realizzazione creativa.

☐ Come cambierebbe la tua vita se riuscissi ad avere gli strumenti giusti per porre fine ai pensieri negativi che ti condizionano e ampliare i tuoi orizzonti verso nuove idee creative alla scoperta del vero te stesso?

Scopri la guida per sviluppare le tue idee più creative, eliminando i pensieri negativi che ti bloccano.

☐ **Qui hai la risposta che stai cercando! Questo libro ti fornirà strategie pratiche per placare la tua mente e prenderne il controllo una volta per tutte. Finalmente hai l'opportunità di accedere alle preziose informazioni che hanno permesso a tantissime persone di stravolgere in meglio la loro vita in modo creativo e pieno di idee nuove per la tua vita. Ed è tutto in questa guida.**

Ecco cosa avrai imparato dopo aver letto questo libro:

- **Riconoscerai quando i tuoi pensieri stanno prendendo il sopravvento, assumendone il controllo**

- **Pensieri negativi: Saprai sfruttare un semplice schema passo dopo passo per eliminare la negatività dalla tua vita**

- La mappa interna: Padroneggerai la tua mappa mentale interiore, scoprirai cos'è esattamente e come può portarti al successo in modo semi automatico e organizzerai le idee nella giusta direzione verso i tuoi obiettivi

- Il potere della mindfulness: Imparerai il più antico strumento di focalizzazione del pensiero, con esercizi pratici per dire per sempre addio ad ansia

- E molto, molto di più...

Smetti di preoccuparti di quello che hai fatto, Inizia a vivere OGGI.

La pace mentale che stai cercando è a distanza di un click...

NON CONTINUARE AD ESSERE SCHIAVO DEI TUOI PENSIERI - Prendi ORA la tua copia

Mente potente :Come Cambiare LA TUA

VITA e VALORIZZARE TE STESSO : Scopri il

tuo potere interiore e vivi la vita che meriti

con esercizi pratici

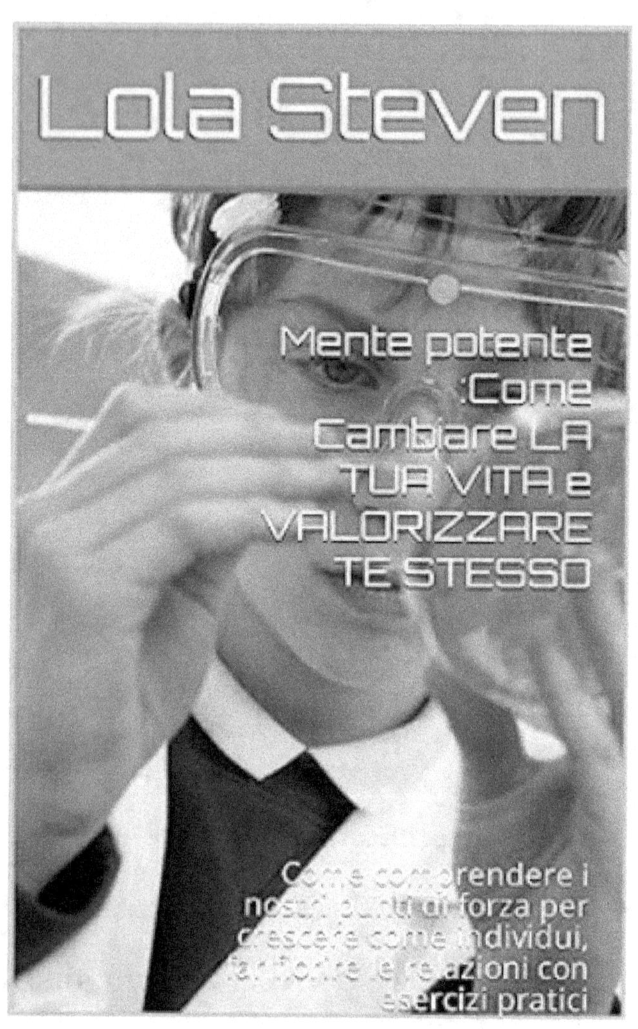

Lola Steven
Mente potente :Come Cambiare LA TUA VITA e VALORIZZARE TE STESSO
Come comprendere i nostri punti di forza per crescere come individui, far fiorire le relazioni con esercizi pratici

Esiste un modo per liberare il tuo potenziale? Vorresti migliorare diversi aspetti della tua vita? Qual è il segreto del talento? Come lo sblocchiamo? Questo lavoro innovativo fornisce ai lettori strumenti che possono utilizzare per massimizzare il potenziale in se stessi e negli altri.

Che tu stia allenando il calcio o insegnando a un bambino a suonare il pianoforte, scrivendo un romanzo o cercando di migliorare il tuo swing da golf, questo libro rivoluzionario ti mostra come far crescere il talento attingendo a un meccanismo cerebrale appena scoperto.

Lola identifica i tre elementi chiave che ti permetteranno di sviluppare i tuoi doni e ottimizzare le tue prestazioni nello sport, nell'arte, nella musica, nella matematica o in qualsiasi altra cosa.

• **Pratica profonda** Tutti sanno che la pratica è la chiave del successo. Quello che tutti non sanno è che specifici tipi di pratica possono aumentare le abilità fino a dieci volte più velocemente rispetto alla pratica convenzionale.

• **Accensione** Abbiamo tutti bisogno di un po' di motivazione per iniziare. Ma cosa separa i veri grandi risultati dal resto del branco? Un livello più alto di impegno – chiamatela passione – nato dai nostri desideri inconsci più profondi e innescato da alcuni segnali primordiali. Capire come funzionano questi segnali può aiutarti ad accendere la passione e catalizzare lo sviluppo delle competenze.

• **Coaching** Quali sono i segreti degli insegnanti, dei formatori e dei coach più efficaci al mondo? Scopri le virtù che consentono a questi "sussurratori di talenti" di alimentare la passione, ispirare una pratica profonda e tirare fuori il meglio dai loro studenti. Questi tre elementi lavorano insieme all'interno del cervello e gli scienziati hanno scoperto che potrebbe essere solo il Santo Graal: il fondamento di tutte le forme di grandezza, da Michelangelo a Michael Jordan. Combinando l'analisi rivelatrice con esempi illuminanti di persone normali che hanno raggiunto la grandezza, questo libro non solo cambierà il modo in cui pensi al talento, ma ti equipaggia per raggiungere il tuo massimo potenziale.

Talento training™ Si articola in :

1. Liberarsi dai condizionamenti, liberare la creatività.

2.Contattare ciò che di unico c'è in te come contributo al mondo.
3.Accedere al nostro sé più autentico per scoprire il proprio potenziale.

Vuoi distinguerti dagli altri e spiccare in mezzo al mare? Farai esercizi pratici sulla storia della tua vita, imparerai a visualizzare i tuoi obiettivi nel modo migliore e nuovo; farai esercizi di simulazione del tuo futuro; imparerai a gestire il denaro; imparerai ad usare la scrittura creativa

Ecco un brano tratto dal libro

La libreria

Pioveva a dirotto in quella fredda e monotona giornata di novembre ed era quasi impossibile vedere attraverso i vetri delle finestre quando, quasi sorta dal nulla, sotto i portici della piazzetta di via Milano comparve una ragazza di bassa statura, grassottella di forse una ventina d'anni. Se un passante l'avesse guardata da vicino, avrebbe scoperto sul suo viso un'espressione sorpresa, dovuta forse agli occhi piuttosto ravvicinati e un sorriso rivelatore di un carattere ancora appena un po' infantile.

I capelli, neri corvini, le ricadevano bagnati sul viso e lo spolverino che indossava era completamente madido di pioggia.

Uscendo come una furia dal luogo dove lavorava pareva sconvolta ma, se lo era, si sarebbe dovuto incolpare il suo capo, un uomo sulla quarantina, isterico e accentratore che aveva il potere di farle perdere l'autocontrollo.

La ragazza, di nome Silvia, una volta sul marciapiede, si era diretta verso una libreria e adesso ,trafelata , si trovava davanti alla vetrina di una libreria, fissando il vuoto.

Ma non durò molto : spalancata la porta quasi con violenza entrò nel negozio attratta dagli scaffali, carichi di libri d' ogni genere.

La lettura era la sua vera passione e per lei nonesisteva nulla di meglio al ondo di un libro per ritrovare serenità e tranquillità.

Stazionava lì, indecisa davanti alla parete tappezzata di libri, quando tra essi ne vide uno che le apparve subito particolare : la copertina era di pelle verde, mail libro era senza titolo.

Senza sapere il perché capì subito, al di là di ogni dubbio, che lei era entrata nel negozio proprio per quel libro, un libro che – lo sentiva intimamente- le apparteneva da sempre.

Lo tolse dallo scaffale e cominciò a sfogliarlo, ma , mentre incuriosita leggeva le prime parole, udì una voce dal suono gentile, delicato. Sorpresa, si guardò intorno per capire da dove provenisse, ma indagare non servì a nulla, perché la voce che aveva udito sorgeva da dentro, nell'anima.

Allora,abbandonate le braccia lungo il corpo, lasciò

che la voce continuasse a sussurrare nella sua mente. "….E' da tanto che ti chiamo, ma tu non mi senti." "Ma com'è possibile?" chiese lei. "Ho sentito le parole provenire dal libro? "…" Sì, sì sono proprio io, il libro!'', esclamò la voce con forza.

Sotto i suoi occhi le pagine incominciarono a svolazzare.

La ragazza era sconvolta dall'esperienza del libro parlante, tuttavia avvertiva la sensazione di essere come cullata da un succedersi di onde serene.

"….Non è difficile comprendere" proseguì la voce" che le azioni malvagie degli uomini esistono perché alla loro base esiste più una conoscenza incompleta del mondo e della realtà circostante, anziché un vero intento malvagio.

Chi agisce con cattiveria nei confronti degli altri lo fa perché non vede alternative e non percepisce gli altri uguali a se stesso e il danno lo compie per proteggersi, non avendo scelte o per l'incapacità di comprendere le altrui prospettive.".

Silvia si irrigidì a quelle parole,ma, nello stesso tempo, non potè fare a meno di rivisitare con quella nuova prospettiva i fatti accaduti in quei giorni al lavoro.

Lavorava come assistente alle vendite in una fabbrica di gioielli di pregio, nota in Italia e all'estero.

Il suo capo era un tipo burbero e arrogante, con un modo di incedere che, agli occhi di chi lo guardava, pareva solo alterigia. Sempre irrigidito, come se fosse costretto a portare lungo la schiena un correttore di legno per la spina dorsale, si muoveva costantemente con atteggiamento irrequieto. Silvia lavorava in uno di quei locali definiti open-space, con altri colleghi, tuttavia il suo capo, immancabilmente, fra tutti, si rivolgeva solo a lei.

Quando era nervoso, lo si capiva da lontano perché spuntava sul suo volto il famoso 'il tic dello gnomo ', affibbiatogli dai dipendenti, consistente in un movimento continuo degli occhi e del naso che li riusciva ad arricciare contemporaneamente. Quando si trovava in questo stato d'animo, l'uomo assumeva un atteggiamento minaccioso, chiedendole dove si trovasse questa o quella pratica, a che punto fosse con i diversi clienti. Una scena che si ripeteva con esasperante continuità mentre lei si domandava quali fossero le sue colpe e che cosa avesse fatto di sbagliato. Eppure era riuscita ad instaurare un buon rapporto con tutti, in ufficio, ma non con il suo capo. Con concentrazione, Silvia stava riflettendo.

" E' interessante ciò che dici, esclamò poi "sembra addirittura che si adatti perfettamente alla mia situazione lavorativa.Puoi spiegarti meglio?" .

"Certamente. Si capisce meglio la prospettiva dell'altro quando è solida la nostra:

bisogna ascoltare se stessi e gli altri per capire il senso della comunicazione senza che il proprio pensiero sia distratto.

La parola ascolto significa rispetto, reciprocità, comprensione.

Se l'altro parla con te è perché vuole comunicare con te; per comprenderlo meglio non devi interromperlo, ma assecondarlo; per capire che cosa pensa, che cosa vuole e perché agisce in un determinato modo devi guardare le cose dal suo punto di vista.Ora se la vuoi ascoltare, ti racconto una storia", concluse il libro.

"Va bene, sentiamo", replicò Silvia.

https://www.amazon.com/Cloud-dog-angry-Illustrated-illustrations-ebook/dp/B0CK8H8W9S/?_encoding=UTF8&pd_rd_w=BGPvn&content-

Cloud the dog is angry: Perfect Illustrated Story Book on how to manage angry for: | Nice plot in rhyme step by step with beautiful illustrations

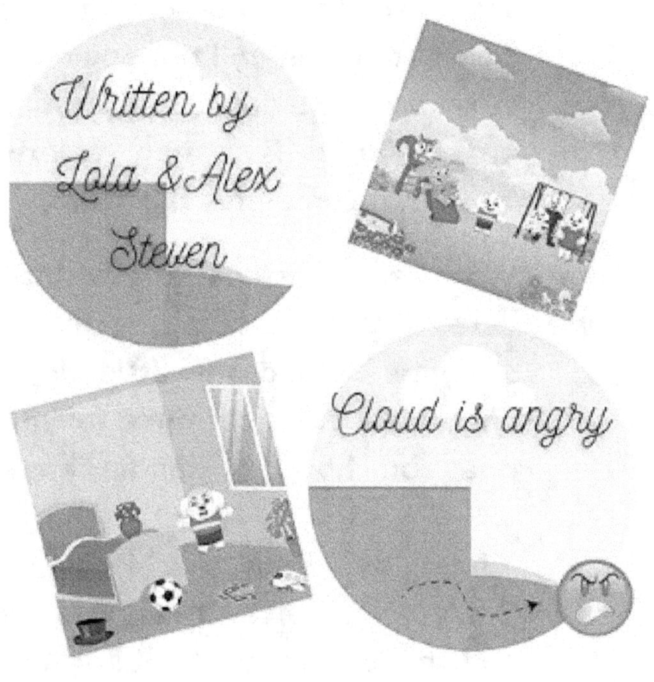
Written by
Lola & Alex Steven
Cloud is angry

Cloud the dog is a story that teaches children how to reduce stress and control anger. Children relate to the angry little dog in this story to calm down and manage anger. Cloud is a new coloring book that completes this story.

With beautiful illustrations and a cute step-by-step rhyming storyline, 'Cloud the little dog is angry' is a great resource for little ones on how to handle anger.

'Cloud the little dog is angry'. Everything, however, annoys him and makes him angry! It's time to learn how to manage emotions... with the approach of Certified Coach Lola Steven and includes:

1. *Easy to follow: Your little one can enjoy this book as a bedtime story, helping him feel safe and happy and strengthening him when he is angry.*

2. *Age-appropriate and engaging content: Using engaging illustrations and easy-to-understand rhyming language, kids will love following Cloud the Little Dog as it shows kids how to manage emotions.*
3. *Inclusive for all toddlers – Cloud the Little Dog has been illustrated as an all-inclusive book from a gender perspective that makes it easy for any child to relate to the plot.*

Product features:

1. *Large size 20x20*
2. *Drawn color illustrations*
3. *28 pages long*
4. *Great writing - perfect for the little ones!*

Reading age: from 3 years.

Children learn to relax, relax and control anger with this fun exercise.

This engaging story calms the mind and relaxes the body so that the child can let go of anger, relax and fall asleep peacefully. Each child has a different emotional maturity, attention span and need. The stories are best suited for children aged 2 to 6 years. Get to know your child better and remember that this is not about the reading level. The focus is on the actual techniques.

Reading age: from 3 years

THANK YOU

I thank all my readers. If you liked the book, go to my website bit.ly/3M6rNgf
To receive news and updates on new books and related events click here and you will be informed

bit.ly/3M6rNgf
If this book has been helpful to you, please leave your review on the left in the amazon link for my book, as it helps to give it more visibility.

Recensisci questo prodotto

Condividi i tuoi pensieri con altri clienti

Scrivi una recensione cliente

Review this product

Share your thoughts with other customers

Write a customer review

And to receive news on Facebook https://www.facebook.com/EmotionVisionDigitalCoaching

Feel free to send me your feedback.

Lola & Dany

INDEX

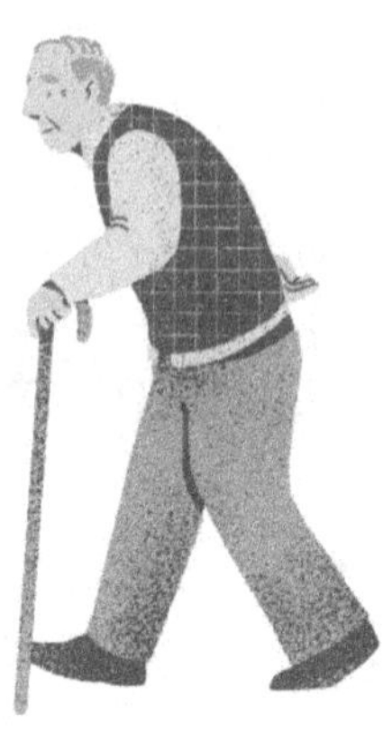

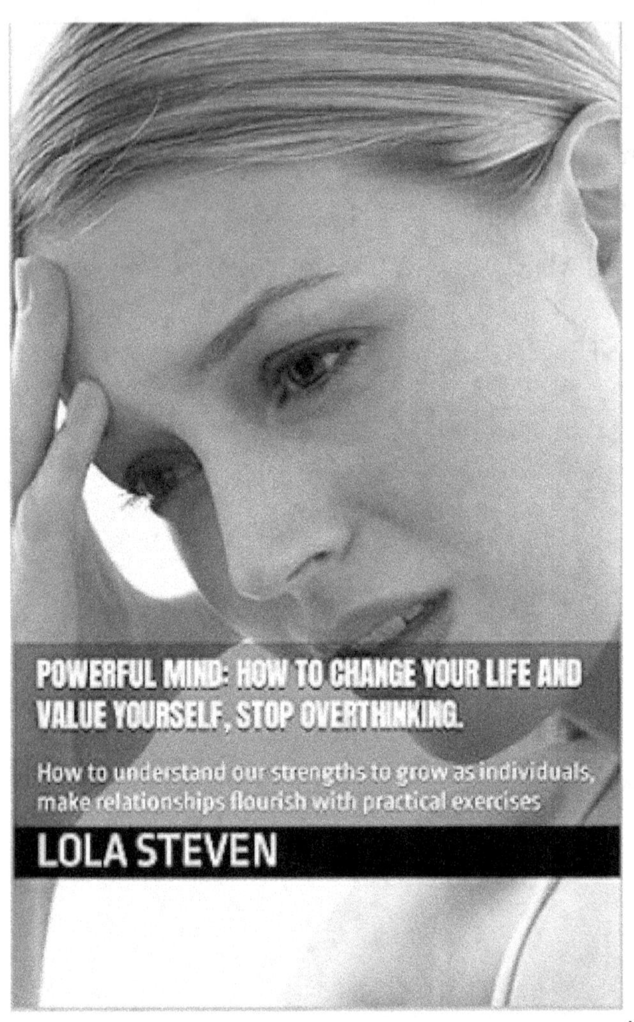

POWERFUL MIND: HOW TO CHANGE YOUR LIFE AND VALUE YOURSELF, STOP OVERTHINKING.
How to understand our strengths to grow as individuals, make relationships flourish with practical exercises
LOLA STEVEN

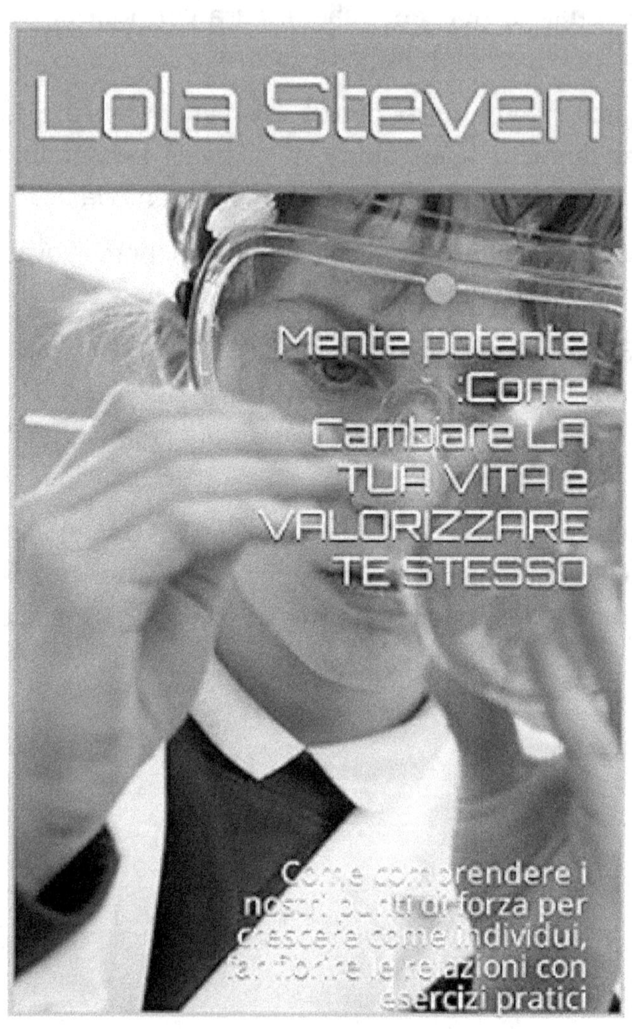

Lola Steven
Mente potente
:Come
Cambiare LA
TUA VITA e
VALORIZZARE
TE STESSO
Come comprendere i
nostri punti di forza per
crescere come individui,
far fiorire le relazioni con
esercizi pratici